Testimonials

I had no energy, was often depressed and tired all the time, yet testing found "nothing wrong." After starting BioSET™ treatments, I saw immediate results. I've lost weight, now run four to six miles a week, work full-time, spend quality time with my children, coach my ten-year-old's soccer team, and feel healthy and happy.

—Connie P.

I've been overweight and had chronic bronchitis my whole life and always got sick over the Christmas holidays. Mainly my allergies have been to food. This year I ate as much of whatever I wanted, yet I did not gain weight, and I didn't get sick. A miracle! Thank you, Dr. Cutler.

—Susan G.

My daughter, Sarah, had severe eczema that covered her face and most of her body. I tried everything from homeopathy to vitamins and herbs. Nothing worked. Sarah's preschool teacher referred me to Dr. Cutler, who evaluated and treated Sarah and taught us how to do home treatments in between office visits. I followed the home-treatment procedure very closely. Sarah's skin is now completely clear, and she has remained free of eczema symptoms for three years. I am so grateful to Dr. Cutler and BioSET™. It has changed our lives. It is so simple, it feels good, and it works.

—Leslie S.

One night I experienced an allergic reaction to shellfish. It was so severe that my tongue swelled up and I had great difficulty swallowing and breathing. Since my very first BioSET™ treatment with Dr. Cutler, I have been able to eat shellfish with no adverse reaction whatsoever.

—*Patricia M.*

Our daughter suffered from allergies since birth. Until she turned thirteen, we were able to keep her condition under control by avoiding the foods that caused her reactions. Then suddenly her allergies flared up, and no matter what we did, they grew worse and worse. Yet after the very first BioSET™ treatment, she felt as if a heavy burden was lifted from her. She couldn't remember ever having felt so good. Within a day, she was able to eat a number of taboo foods with absolutely no allergic reaction. The stunning success of BioSET™ brought our daughter from a crippling, lifelong disability to a reasonably normal life in a matter of weeks.

—*J. Chapman*

Eight months ago, I traveled to California to see Dr. Ellen Cutler. I was extremely ill and periodically experienced episodes of loss of consciousness up to two hours. I came to realize that there was not much left that I could eat without having a reaction. After the first two weeks of treatments, I could eat a wide variety of foods. I also felt and looked much better, and a nice extra—my hair became thicker. I'm back for three more weeks of treatments. I only wish that everyone who is having allergy problems could experience BioSET™ treatment.

—*Donna B.*

I first visited Dr. Cutler's clinic last August for my asthma. The good news is that this allergy season, I did not have a single asthma attack for the first time in twenty years!

—*Dean M.*

THE
FOOD
ALLERGY
CURE

Also by Dr. Ellen Cutler

Winning the War Against Asthma & Allergies

Winning the War Against Immune Disorders & Allergies

THE FOOD ALLERGY CURE

A New Solution to Food Cravings,
Obesity, Depression, Headaches,
Arthritis, and Fatigue

DR. ELLEN W. CUTLER

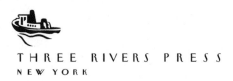

THREE RIVERS PRESS
NEW YORK

Published by Three Rivers Press, New York, New York.
Member of the Crown Publishing Group, a division of Random House, Inc.

www.randomhouse.com

THREE RIVERS PRESS and the Tugboat design are registered trademarks of Random House, Inc.

Originally published in hardcover by Harmony Books, a division of Random House, Inc., New York, in 2001.

Printed in the United States of America

Design by Meryl Sussman Levavi/Digitext

Illustrations by Jennifer Harper

Library of Congress Cataloging-in-Publication Data

Cutler, Ellen W.
    The food allergy cure / by Ellen Cutler.—1st ed.
        p. cm.
    Includes bibliographical references.
    1. Food allergy—Alternative treatment.   2. Applied kinesiology.   3. Chiropractic.
4. Acupressure. I. Title.
RC596 .C88 2001
616.97'506—dc21

                                                                                00-058084

ISBN 0-609-80900-8

10   9   8   7   6   5   4   3   2   1

First Paperback Revised Edition

The Food Allergy Cure is dedicated to all the BioSET™ practitioners who trust and support me each and every day in my passion to restore optimal health to the world, by using natural medicine.

Acknowledgments

There are many people to thank, including my loving family, who continuously support me in my passion as a healer, lecturer, and author. I love them very much, and they are with me in my heart and soul with every word I write. Thank you, Aaron and Gabrielle.

I express my sincere gratitude to:

Joy Parker and Nancy Faass, my guardian angels, who skillfully, patiently, and brilliantly edited *The Food Allergy Cure*. They are true artists, and I feel they have become a part of my family forever.

My other guardian angel, my assistant, without whom I could never have completed this manuscript. She has helped me take BioSET™ to another level. Her expert assistance, maturity, and precision astonish me each and every day we work together. Thank you, Agnes Liebhardt, for your love, faith, and undying support.

My literary agent, Bonnie Solow, who saw the promise of my work and guided and instructed me as I gained strength and maturity as an author and leader in my field.

Patricia Gift and Carrie Thornton, my editors at Harmony Books and

Three Rivers Press, whose genius, vision, intuition, and passion turned the manuscript into the complete, rich, informative, and important composition I believe it has now become. Thank you, Patty and Carrie, for believing in me.

Gary Kaplan, our business manager, whose selfless and heartwarming efforts on behalf of BioSET™ are gratefully acknowledged.

Brent Ottley—a friend, fellow lecturer, and true master in his field as an acupuncturist, writer, and energetic healer—who brilliantly helped research, write, and edit *The Food Allergy Cure.* His attention to detail and commitment to the truth gave a deeper vision and dimension to this document.

Deborah Cutler, D.C., my sister-in-law, who has brought BioSET™ to the community and stands strong as a leader in the field of natural healing.

Bart Stein, L.Ac., who graciously helped in solidifying the at-home allergy elimination technique. Thank you, Bart, for your support and your guidance.

Lynn Greaves at Enzymes Incorporated, who had faith in me and shared my vision—which enabled the creation of the highest-grade vegetarian enzymes on the market today.

I am also grateful to:

My family and friends, including Seymour and Miriam Wagner, Dr. Ira Wagner, and Thekla Wagner for their invaluable love and support.

Deborah Santana, who is my dearest friend. She is always there for me. Her emotional and spiritual presence is a true and sacred healing tool that I will always honor and treasure.

Shelley Campbell, who is not only my daughter's friend and caretaker but also my dear friend. Without her, this manuscript could never have been completed. She watches over my family so I can write, care for my patients, and have the time and ability to succeed as a healer, author, and leader in the health field.

Molly Kimball, who created these yummy recipes and meal plans. Her artistry will be an important help for my readers.

Contents

THE
FOOD
ALLERGY
CURE

1

A New Approach to Food Allergies

THE HAZARDS OF HIDDEN FOOD ALLERGIES

Are you one of the more than ninety million Americans suffering from allergies? Or are you one of those who are unaware that they have allergies because the health symptoms seem totally unrelated? Typically we think of allergies as the cause of sniffles and sneezes, even sinus conditions and headaches. Yet there are many other conditions we rarely associate with allergies, ranging from hyperactivity to chronic fatigue. In fact, fatigue is one of the main characteristics of allergies. Other disorders linked to allergies include many types of chronic skin conditions, digestive illness, and mood disorders, including depression.

Most people who realize that allergies are causing their symptoms view them as something they must learn to live with. They usually hold little hope for recovery, beyond temporary relief through medication. This resignation reflects the widespread belief that allergies are incurable. Yet over the past twenty years, I have successfully treated thousands of sufferers. If you suspect that allergies are a factor in your health, I offer encouragement. In most cases, they can be eliminated.

Allergies seem minor compared to diseases such as cancer. Although allergies are rarely life-threatening, they place a drain on the immune system as a constant source of stress. Allergic reactions usually cause irritation. Whenever irritation or inflammation is present for an extended period of time, the body's cells and tissues are gradually damaged. Over time, these changes can develop into identifiable diseases such as arthritis or asthma. At that point, the damage may be irreversible. In the case of rheumatoid arthritis, even simple movements become painful, and the joints and bones eventually distort. When asthmatic reactions occur, every breath becomes a struggle, and the lung tissue is often affected. Yet long before this damage is evident, there is inflammation. Both arthritis and asthma are often linked to allergies and related inflammation. They represent only two examples of the dangerous effects of hidden allergies.

If you have allergies, you may find yourself going to great lengths to find relief from your symptoms. Perhaps you've tried complicated or austere diets. You may have tried to relieve your symptoms with medications that can have unpleasant side effects, including mood swings, headaches, or fluid retention. You may experience even more serious long-term consequences, such as suppression of the immune system or osteoporosis. A small number of allergy patients develop so many sensitivities that they become virtual shut-ins, unable to function in normal society. Treatment may be expensive, complex, and inconvenient. If you are an allergy sufferer, you may find yourself adapting to your condition with resignation, attempting to avoid the sources that provoke your symptoms. Most people who face these challenges agree that allergies almost always compromise health and quality of life.

A NEW METHOD OF ALLERGY TREATMENT

There is now an effective technique for treating allergies of any kind. Thousands of patients across the country and worldwide have found that this method permanently eliminates allergies. So the goal of this book is not to avoid allergenic foods. Rather, it introduces a system for *eliminating* allergies: BioSET™, which can neutralize the body's allergic response to foods and other substances.

A NATURAL SYSTEM OF HEALING

BioSET™ effectively treats allergies and many related health conditions. It is based on an innovative allergy treatment using acupressure. The method is used in combination with good nutrition, enzyme therapy, and detoxification. These therapies remove the stressors on the immune system to restore health and natural vitality.

BioSET™ focuses on three key areas:

1. A unique acupressure technique that eliminates allergies and sensitivities, often permanently
2. Nutritional evaluation and the use of enzymes to correct deficiencies and improve digestion and function
3. Purifying and detoxifying the body through homeopathic remedies and lifestyle therapies

BioSET™ is gaining scientific credibility and grateful adherents around the world. Over the past ten years, I have treated thousands of patients who have experienced total relief from their allergy symptoms. This approach has also been successful for tens of thousands more around the world who have been treated by practitioners I have trained.

THE DEVELOPMENT OF BIOSET™

The BioSET™ system was developed through years of observation in clinical practice and ongoing evaluation of a wide range of allergy therapies. It also grew out of my own search for healing and transformation. In addition, the therapies incorporate the experience of other health care professionals and patients. I personally suffered from food allergies for many years. Throughout my education in chiropractic college and years of postgraduate training, I explored every reasonable treatment option. After studying enzyme therapy with the respected naturopathic physician Bernard Jensen, I began taking digestive enzymes. Many of my symptoms disappeared, yet I still felt fatigued and depressed after eating certain foods. Once I developed my own practice, I continued to explore methods and products that might alleviate my allergies and those of my patients.

I had a major breakthrough when I learned of the work of an acupuncturist who had discovered a technique for evaluating and treating allergies. I observed her work and found her success rate impressive. Soon I began referring my most difficult patients to her. One of the first was a woman who suffered from severe chronic nasal congestion and shortness of breath. Her evaluation indicated allergies to dust, mold, pollen, cat dander, certain vitamins, and some fruits and vegetables. After a series of acupuncture treatments for these allergens, the patient was completely free of her symptoms.

I was so impressed that I began referring more patients to the acupuncturist, and I also went for treatment myself. Initially she treated me for allergies to various food groups, including egg whites, milk, and sugar. I was especially sensitive to sugar, which caused me headaches and depression. After treatment, I no longer reacted negatively to sugar. Not only was I symptom-free, but my cravings for sweets had vanished as well. I also felt a tremendous increase in energy. The acupuncturist continued treating me for other food allergies, including grains and dairy products. By the time the treatments were completed, I no longer had to limit my food intake in any way. I was allergy-free.

I began to integrate these methods into my clinical practice and, over time, evolved an advanced system of healing. This approach incorporates acupressure and traditional Chinese medicine with applied immunology and state-of-the-art nutrition. Equally important, this simple and effective system provides tools that anyone can use to maintain optimal health.

HOW TO USE THIS BOOK

The early chapters describe the basic ideas behind the BioSET™ technique and the conditions it benefits. I provide step-by-step instructions for each phase of home allergy treatment, including testing methods. It also explains the basics of enzyme therapy and detoxification. Comprehensive tables in the back of the book allow you to easily correlate symptoms with foods.

GENTLE ACUPRESSURE

BioSET™ allergy treatment involves the use of acupressure—gentle stimulation of specific points on the body (acupoints) using the fingertips. Some forms of this technique can be learned by anyone and used in home treatment, described in chapter 8. Complex cases are best addressed by a trained practitioner. BioSET™ is also effective for allergies to environmental substances such as pollen, dust, animal dander, or chemicals.

Acupressure can be provided while the subject is fully clothed. The most important acupoints are located along either side of the backbone. Gentle stimulation can have a profound effect, benefiting the immune system and other areas of the body. In traditional Chinese medicine, these points are described as "association points" because they are associated with the body's flow of energy. Gently massaging the association points has been found to "reprogram" the body's response to a food or substance that triggers an allergy.

DETOXIFICATION

Healing from food allergies also means learning simple methods to purify and detoxify. Since toxicity is an inescapable part of life in the industrial world, we need to recognize and minimize toxic exposure whenever possible. It is also important to clear accumulated toxins by incorporating detoxification into our daily lives. Even small changes in lifestyle can have beneficial effects. Chapter 9 offers practical suggestions for simple home practice.

Detoxification aids the function of your immune system by clearing toxins from the cells and tissues, especially the digestive tract, skin, and lungs. Your immune function protects your body from invasion by microbes and tumor cells. However, immune performance is reduced whenever there is toxicity, poor digestion, or inflammation from allergies. These problems can overwhelm the system, causing illness. By minimizing toxins, you lighten the burden on the immune system and its network of defenses. So detoxification is a primary and natural beginning to any healing process. Immediate, practical approaches to detoxification include:

- Drinking plenty of water
- Wise use of juicing and fasting
- Breathing techniques
- Dry-skin brushing
- Detoxifying baths and saunas
- Cleansing the digestive tract
- Homeopathic remedies for detoxification
- Massage

It is also important to develop a long-term program that enables the body to periodically detoxify by:

- Improving the way we eat
- Minimizing foods that do not support our health
- Exercising regularly
- Decompressing from emotional trauma and stress
- Reducing toxic exposures

ENZYME THERAPY

All living organisms depend on enzymes. They are required in more than 150,000 biochemical reactions in the body, particularly those involving the digestion of food and the delivery of nutrients throughout the system.

Enzymes can be divided into three major categories: metabolic enzymes, digestive enzymes, and natural enzymes in the foods we eat. Digestive enzymes are secreted in the mouth, the stomach, the pancreas, and the small intestine. These enzymes are vital for the proper digestion of everything we eat.

Simply stated, all fruits and vegetables contain natural enzymes that help us digest them. The problem with the modern diet is that these enzymes are destroyed by overcooking, canning, and other forms of food processing. Even if we get enough enzymes, we often cannot utilize them if we don't chew our food well, a minimum of thirty times. If you try chewing each bite thirty times, you'll soon realize that you may be eating your food far too fast. Our rapidly paced lifestyle has destroyed the luxury of savoring our food so that it can be fully digested in the process. Enzymes are a right and natural cure for many digestive problems. By improving digestion, some allergy symptoms are also improved or eliminated. Chapter 10 considers the important role of digestive enzymes and how to incorporate them into your own diet.

WHEN TO USE HOME TREATMENT AND WHEN TO SEE A PRACTITIONER

Severe allergies should always be treated by a health care practitioner, ideally one with extensive BioSET™ training. BioSET™ self-care is not a substitute for treatment by an expert practitioner, in the same sense that reading a medical textbook can provide a better understanding of various conditions yet does not make one a doctor.

If your allergies put you at risk for shock (anaphylaxis), or if you have ever had one of these reactions, do not attempt to self-treat. Seek expert medical care.

WHO BENEFITS FROM HOME TREATMENT

Patients who seem to respond the best to self-care are those with simple food allergies. If you have a complex medical condition, see a health care practitioner. BioSET™ self-treatment is most appropriate:

- *If you have clearly identified allergies, but they aren't regarded as life-threatening.* Those who have had a scratch test or a medical diagnosis that points to specific allergens tend to be good candidates for home treatment.
- *If you have mild to moderate symptoms.* People with simple food allergies are less likely to run into problems with home treatment.
- *If you grasp the concept.* People who understand and feel comfortable with the technique tend to do well with this approach.

WHEN TO SEE A PRACTITIONER

If you want coaching on the use of BioSET™, it can be helpful to work under the supervision of a trained practitioner. You still have the option of using some self-treatment; practitioners usually offer patients the opportunity to become involved in their own care.

- *If you have serious or long-term illness.* People with significant illness or severe allergies require the supervision of a practitioner. It is also important to differentiate allergies from other health problems. For example, a patient who has nasal stuffiness and congestion on only one side may have an allergy, but he could also be dealing with a polyp, tumor, or some other serious underlying problem.

Most patients who are quite ill tend to benefit from home care because they may need additional treatments between appointments. This makes it possible to increase the frequency of allergy clearing, since it usually is not practical to have office visits every day or two. The practitioner can supervise and monitor patient efforts:

- *When your allergies are complex.* Patients can self-treat for some simple food allergens. The practitioner is trained to address complex aspects of care:
  —*Allergies involving the body's biochemistry and hormonal systems*

—*Multiple food allergies* in which the interaction of two or more foods or substances together trigger allergic symptoms

—*Multiple chemical sensitivities,* conditions such as environmental allergies or chronic fatigue syndrome that often require specialized expertise to treat

—*Cross-reacting allergies,* which reflect the presence of both allergies and reactivity involving specific acupoints or meridians: these require skill to diagnose and treat, and they should be cleared only by a practitioner

- *If you live far from a practitioner.* BioSET™ practitioners often make it a point to teach self-care techniques to patients who must travel a long distance to receive treatment.

WORKING WITH YOUR PRACTITIONER

The treatments provided by practitioners resemble those described in this book but are more sophisticated and take into account other factors of the patient's health. Practitioners receive in-depth training in order to perform this therapy effectively.

BioSET™ practitioners find that patients can become more confident in providing self-care once they have received several office treatments. After experiencing gentle acupressure, a patient can use this technique at home and then return to the practitioner's office every few weeks to be checked for cleared allergies. At that time, the practitioner will also provide treatment for more complex allergy conditions beyond the scope of self-care.

I would like to emphasize that it is important that patients with major health issues be checked by a BioSET™ provider. When these patients self-treat without supervision, they may experience long-term treatment failures with regard to their allergies.

As with any other skill, you will probably find that you gradually develop greater facility in performing the treatment. Often practitioners encourage patients to come in every week or two to be rechecked for allergy clearings performed at home. Using this approach, it is possible to clear five or six food allergies a week through self-care. Frequently only one or two of the allergens need to be retreated. For patients with complex conditions, working with a BioSET™ practitioner provides the best of both worlds.

WHEN TO SEE A PRACTITIONER IF YOU ARE USING HOME TREATMENT

At what point do you seek out a practitioner?

- *If the treatments have had no effect.* If you find that three to four self-care treatments have had no effect, the problem may be too complex to be addressed through home care. You might also need assistance in perfecting the technique and may find it helpful to review the home treatment by watching the video *Creating Wellness,* available from the BioSET™ Institute (see the appendix).
- *If your allergies improve and then worsen.* When you experience some improvement but the benefit is not sustained, see a practitioner. A thorough series of BioSET™ treatments usually resolves allergies permanently. Remember, you still have the option of providing the home treatments. However, you will also receive evaluation, professional treatment, and monitoring. When patients and practitioners work together, the treatment will proceed faster, save time and money, and involve patients in the process.

HEALTH SCREENING QUESTIONNAIRE (HSQ)

This questionnaire can be used as a tool to measure the severity of your symptoms and assess the need for a visit to a health care practitioner. The test is a reliable evaluation tool, developed and validated by a university research team. At this point, the HSQ has been used worldwide in more than two hundred thousand health assessments.

When you take the test, take your time and be honest with yourself. Report everything, no matter how insignificant. You may even want to give yourself two scores, to reflect your highs and lows. To do this, make two columns—one for good days and one for bad days. Rate each of the following symptoms based on your typical experience.

Point Scale:

0 = Never or almost never have the symptom
1 = Occasionally have it, effect is not severe
2 = Occasionally have it, effect is severe
3 = Frequently have it, effect is not severe
4 = Frequently have it, effect is severe

HEAD

____ Headaches
____ Faintness
____ Dizziness
____ Insomnia   Total ____

EYES

____ Watery or itchy eyes
____ Swollen, reddened, or sticky eyelids
____ Bags or dark circles under eyes
____ Blurred or tunnel vision
      (does not include near- or farsightedness)   Total ____

EARS

____ Itchy ears
____ Earaches, ear infections
____ Drainage from ear
____ Ringing in ears, hearing loss   Total ____

NOSE

____ Stuffy nose
____ Sinus problems
____ Hay fever
____ Sneezing attacks
____ Excessive mucus   Total ____

MOUTH/THROAT

____ Chronic coughing
____ Gagging, frequent need to clear throat
____ Sore throat, hoarseness, loss of voice
____ Swollen or discolored tongue, gums, lips
____ Canker sores   Total ____

SKIN

____ Acne
____ Hives, rashes, dry skin
____ Hair loss
____ Flushing, hot flashes
____ Excessive sweating   Total ____

HEART	____ Irregular or skipped heartbeat	
	____ Rapid or pounding heartbeat	
	____ Chest pain	Total ____

LUNGS	____ Chest congestion	
	____ Asthma, bronchitis	
	____ Shortness of breath	
	____ Difficulty breathing	Total ____

DIGESTIVE TRACT	____ Nausea, vomiting	
	____ Diarrhea	
	____ Constipation	
	____ Bloated feeling	
	____ Heartburn	
	____ Intestinal/stomach pain	Total ____

JOINTS/MUSCLES	____ Pain or aches in joints	
	____ Arthritis	
	____ Stiffness or limitation of movement	
	____ Pain or aches in muscles	
	____ Feeling of weakness or tiredness	Total ____

WEIGHT	____ Binge eating/drinking	
	____ Craving certain foods	
	____ Excessive weight	
	____ Compulsive eating	
	____ Water retention	
	____ Underweight	Total ____

ENERGY/ACTIVITY	____ Fatigue, sluggishness	
	____ Apathy, lethargy	
	____ Hyperactivity	
	____ Restlessness	Total ____

MIND	____ Poor memory	
	____ Confusion, poor comprehension	
	____ Poor concentration	
	____ Poor physical coordination	
	____ Difficulty in making decisions	
	____ Stuttering or stammering	

	____ Slurred speech	
	____ Learning disabilities	Total ____
EMOTIONS	____ Mood swings	
	____ Anxiety, fear, nervousness	
	____ Anger, irritability, aggressiveness	
	____ Depression	Total ____
OTHER SYMPTOMS	____ Frequent or urgent urination	
	____ Genital itch or discharge	
	____ Frequent illness	Total ____
		TOTAL SCORE ____

The Health Screening Questionnaire is adapted with permission from the Immuno Symptom Checklist (ISC), ⊕ 1988 by Immuno Laboratories, Inc., Fort Lauderdale, FL, 800-231-9197. The ISC has been used by more than two hundred thousand patients and their physicians worldwide to assist in the evaluation of food allergies and IgG-mediated "delayed" food sensitivities.

INTERPRETING YOUR SCORE

The total score can indicate the overall severity of your symptoms, while the individual sections can highlight specific problem areas. A score of 50 or greater may reflect the possibility of food allergies. Unfortunately, food allergies are often difficult to diagnose. Some can cause a direct response in the body, while others cause a delayed reaction and are therefore harder to detect. If you scored 75 or greater, seriously consider seeking the assistance of a BioSET™ practitioner or other health care professional in your area.

2

What Is an Allergy?

ANNA'S STORY

Anna, a three-year-old girl who was brought to see me, had eczema so severe that the only part of her body clear of any outbreak was her face. Her parents had tried many healing modalities, including homeopathy, vitamins, and creams, with no success. Finally a family mentioned that Anna might have food allergies and that they should inquire into this area. I was amazed that no doctor had even brought up this possibility, as many physicians have become aware of the possible correlation between food sensitivities and skin eruptions and would normally perform some of the standard testing for food allergies.

When Anna's parents went back to their physician and asked that she be tested for food allergies, the only things that came up positive were mold and dust—no food sensitivities. Anna's parents were not satisfied with this conclusion and felt the need to obtain a second opinion. They saw evidence in Anna's daily life that she might have food allergies. For example, they told me that after she ate eggs Anna would scratch till she bled, and cry excessively during her sleep. Searching the Internet for information about allergies, eczema, and treatments led them to my Web site and consequently to my office.

I was able to test Anna for many of her daily food items, and after we got the results her parents were able to keep her away from those foods to which she was allergic until we could clear them with the BioSET™ allergy elimination technique. I offered to teach Anna's parents the technique so that they themselves could begin clearing food allergies; considering that they lived quite a distance from my clinic, with no other BioSET™ practitioner around, I felt this would be wise.

Two weeks later, when Anna walked in the front door of my clinic and saw me standing in the hallway, she ran up to me and hugged my legs. "How is she?" I asked her parents.

Before they could answer, she replied, "I don't scratch anymore—look at my arms." When she raised the right sleeve of her T-shirt to show me her upper arm, I could see that there was no eczema.

Her parents told me that there was no more scratching, no more crying at night, and therefore some very good sleep for all. They continued, "If it hadn't been for your allergy tests, we never would have known what was bothering our little girl, and she would have continued suffering. And we know we can look forward to your clearing these allergies so that she doesn't need to be deprived of these foods for much longer. We're ready to learn how to help her."

Anna's parents continued to eliminate their daughter's allergies at home through the BioSET™ allergy elimination technique I had taught them, and Anna can now eat a wide variety of foods with no reactions.

ELIMINATING FOOD ALLERGIES

Clinical studies of the BioSET™ allergy elimination technique have proven it to be the most effective, easiest, and fastest treatment for the elimination of allergies. To understand how BioSET™ works, it is useful to think of the body as an organism through which electromagnetic energy flows along invisible pathways. According to Chinese medicine, this electromagnetic energy in our bodies, which it calls chi, manifests as lines of force that run near the body's surface, then pass into our internal organs. These lines of force are called meridians. The amount of energy conducted through our acupuncture meridians can be measured and recorded. This is done either through muscle testing or with an electrical device that measures the electrical properties of the body's meridians and indicates whether they are balanced, stressed, weakened, or blocked. Acupuncturists employ a variety of techniques to eliminate imbalances or blockages in the natural flow of energy through the body. BioSET™ uses tools drawn from acupuncture, chiropractic, and kinesiology to locate and remove blockages in the electromagnetic pathways that are specifically related to allergens.

WHY ALLERGIC REACTIONS TAKE PLACE

When an allergen enters the body, there is a clash between the energy field of the allergen and the energy field of the allergy sufferer. This sets off a chain reaction in the body. First the immune system makes a concerted effort to protect the body from a substance it perceives as harmful by identifying the allergen and sending an alert throughout the body via messenger chemicals. The immune system responds by producing antibodies that aid in the destruction of the substance, blocking the allergen from damaging the system. Technically, this occurrence is called an antigen-antibody bond, and it is the immune system's defense against foreign matter or germs.

When any substance perceived as a foreign agent enters the body, whether it is ingested, inhaled, touched, or injected, the body defends itself with white blood cells such as T cells, B cells, as well as antibodies. Antibodies are minute proteins that function as artillery, bombarding germs or allergenic food particles. This type of immune reaction causes the release of substances such as histamines from the cells into the bloodstream. These substances are called immune mediators and are part of the process of tissue inflammation in the body, which is what commonly creates those swollen, red eyes we see in allergy sufferers. These immune responses may also cause blockages in the body's electromagnetic energy pathways. So the body's reaction to allergens can produce any number of symptoms, from constricted sinuses, throat, or breathing passages, to vomiting, diarrhea, or watery eyes.

The operation of the body's immune system is complex. We still do not fully understand how a substance triggers, regulates, or stops an immune response. Nor do we really understand why some individuals are allergic to cashews and others to shrimp or shellfish. Genetics plays a role in this, as do stress, poor digestion, environmental toxicity, and poor nutrition. I have named this the *load phenomenon,* based on the idea that we can go for years without being allergic to something. Then one day, when our emotional and physical stresses increase to a certain point, we suddenly have a burden great enough to tip the balance within our body. Common physical stresses include menopausal changes and poor dietary habits.

Whenever energy blockages occur in the body, health problems inevitably result. The symptoms produced by such blockages include bodily aches and pains, sore throats, fever, chills, painful lymph nodes, weakness, extreme fatigue, headaches, sleep disturbances, irritability, confusion, depression, forgetfulness, burning sensations in the body, frequent urination, crying spells, sores in the mouth, indigestion, bloating, water retention, or even suicidal behavior and death. But virtually any symptom can be the result of a blockage caused by an allergen.

Symptoms vary depending on the meridian along which the energy blockage occurs. For instance, if the energy flow is blocked in the meridian that leads to the lung and large intestine, a person might suffer from severe respiratory distress, asthma, chills, sinus problems, constipation, or diarrhea. If the blockage is in the kidney meridian, the person may suffer from water retention or frequent urination. A blockage in the energy flow of the gallbladder meridian may produce pain and swelling in the breast, pain in the rib and chest muscles, abdominal cramping, heavy menstrual bleeding, severe mood swings, aggressive behavior, or anger. Energy blockages in the heart meridians can cause heart palpitations, cardiac arrhythmia, insomnia, dry mouth, heavy sensations in the chest, night sweats, fatigue, or insecurity.

BioSET™ practitioners use chiropractic spinal techniques to stimulate acupressure points connected to each meridian. If a blockage affects a certain meridian, the practitioner stimulates the acupressure point along the spine connected to that meridian. For example, a wheat allergy can cause a blockage in the lung meridian and can result in breathing difficulties. To treat a wheat allergy, a BioSET™ practitioner stimulates the acupressure points along the spine that are related to the lungs while the patient holds the particular allergen, in this case wheat. Soon after the treatment is completed, the person will no longer be sensitive to wheat. Through the BioSET™ technique, the body's allergy complexes can literally be reprogrammed, one allergen at a time.

TWO CASE STUDIES IN THE TREATMENT OF FOOD ALLERGIES

Over the years I have been practicing as an allergy specialist, I have encountered amazing and dramatic results in the patients who have come to me for help. I have learned that any symptom can be the result of food allergies. I have also seen firsthand that the BioSET™ treatment can often cure conditions that other medical treatments could not. Here are two significant examples.

✑ BETSY'S STORY

Betsy, eighty-one, had been diagnosed with polymyalgia rheumatica (PMR) eight years before she first came to see me in 1996. PMR is characterized by achiness in the muscles of the neck, shoulders, or hips, especially in the morning. Patients feel stiff all over and have trouble getting out of the bed. This disease can strike without warning and can be accompanied by headaches, hearing difficulties, and a persistent cough. Although the cause is uncertain, the standard treatment is corticosteroids.

Betsy experienced severe pain in her shoulder and arms that would wake her up frequently throughout the night. For the past three years she had been taking prednisone, which gave her some relief. But as time went on, she began to develop allergies to a number of foods, including dairy products, grains, and alcohol. Among her symptoms were diarrhea, chronic sinus congestion, and hypoglycemia. In fact, she needed to eat constantly to avoid feeling lethargic or faint. Once a highly energetic woman, Betsy was slowed down by the allergies and the PMR. Betsy decided to stop taking prednisone, even though it lessened her pain, because of its many side effects, which can include osteoporosis (diminished bone density) and allergies.

When I performed a complete allergy assessment, it revealed that Betsy was allergic to minerals, especially calcium and magnesium. Treatment with the BioSET™ allergy elimination technique for calcium and magnesium often proves helpful in relieving the joint pain associated with rheumatoid arthritis, osteoarthritis, and fibromyalgia, and I was hoping that Betsy might respond to this treatment as well. She also proved to be allergic to all calcium- and magnesium-rich foods, such as milk, cheese, soybeans, grains, green leafy vegetables, fruits, and berries.

After describing the technique to her and treating her for her calcium and magnesium allergies, I was gratified to see that Betsy's shoulder and arm pain completely disappeared for the first time since 1988. Her stamina returned, and she was able to sleep all night without interruption. In addition, she could now take calcium and magnesium supplements, which used to make her sick to her stomach, and eat all of the above foods without any problem. It was one of the most dramatic and exciting improvements I have ever seen.

ᴥ ERIC'S STORY

Eric, five years old, was brought by his mother to my office late one afternoon. Eric had on dark sunglasses and a large baseball cap that he wore low on his forehead. He walked with stooped shoulders, like a ninety-year-old man with arthritis. My receptionist brought him back to our "kids' room," where I observed him for a while.

As soon as he entered the room, he shut off the light and sat cross-legged on the floor, head down, eyes staring at the ground. Was he autistic? I wondered! Or was he dressing up in a costume? Both my guesses were wrong. His mother, Joan, described the problem to me. Evidently Eric was extremely sensitive to light. Even when inside a building on a cloudy day, he could not function without wearing sunglasses. He was continually laughed at in school, and his teachers were very upset at what they called his "shenanigans." Because of his sensitivity, he was not able to play any sports, and he was depressed.

When I first tried to talk to Eric, he was unresponsive and teary. Although he would not remove his shades or his cap or let me see into his eyes, I could hear it in his voice. How was I to begin to help him? I stepped out of the room for a moment and took a deep breath.

Then I walked back into the kids' room and sat down cross-legged on the floor. I was barely able to engage his eyes, but nonetheless, I spoke to Eric from the heart. I told him that I really did not understand exactly how he felt but that a lot of sick children who came to see

(continued)

me got well. "Maybe you can get well," I said. "I can't promise it, but I think your eyes might be so sensitive because you are allergic to a food."

Eric thought for a moment, lifted up his head, looked me in the eyes, and took off his hat. Shortly afterward he removed his glasses. His eyes were almost fully closed, severely reddened, and obviously very painful. I had to help this child.

I began to do some allergy testing and found that Eric was allergic to many foods. Joan told me that Eric had tried a variety of different treatments, including homeopathy, steroids, antihistamines, herbs, and vitamins. Some were more successful than others, but only for short periods of time.

We set up a series of twice-weekly treatments for Eric and began working on eliminating his allergies. Initially there was no real improvement in his condition, although Eric did begin to feel more comfortable with me and enjoyed coming into the office. BioSET™ allergy treatments are a pleasant experience, almost like a massage. Since at that point in time my own daughter was five, I was able to relate to Eric very well. We hit it off, and I must say I looked forward to seeing this little boy.

The Friday afternoon arrived when we had planned to treat Eric for sugars. As he walked into my office holding on to his mother, I immediately noticed that his demeanor had changed; he seemed withdrawn. What had happened? I asked Joan about the problem.

"Well," she replied, "he didn't want to be treated for sugars."

As I was about to ask her why this was a problem, I suddenly realized that Eric was addicted to sugar—and that this could be a crucial turning point in his treatment. I went ahead and gave Eric the BioSET™ treatment for sugars. He didn't even look at me or acknowledge me that day. He just grunted and let me work on him. I respected his uneasiness.

The following Tuesday afternoon, the day of Eric's next appointment, I spotted a strange boy walking around the corner of my office into the kids' room. I usually don't see new clients at the end of the day, but I thought that maybe this was an emergency. When I asked my receptionist who this person was, she told me it was Eric.

I could hardly believe what she was saying. I ran into the kids' room and looked at Eric. He was wearing neither the sunglasses nor his cap, and he looked straight into my eyes and did not squint. Unaware of my shock, he began to talk to me about Beanie Babies.

When I glanced at his mother, she was smiling. She told me that within two hours of receiving the BioSET™ treatment for sugars, Eric had removed his glasses and hat and had not put them on since. It was a miracle.

I was happy but tried to be a little conservative. "Let's wait a few more weeks to see if his condition stays improved. Meanwhile, we'll continue treating him for his other food allergies."

That same day Joan revealed to me what she had failed to mention earlier: Her husband, Eric's father, is a diabetic. As compensation for his own inability to eat sugar, he would offer Eric sugar constantly. For this reason, Eric had slowly become addicted to sugar, so much so that sugary foods would often substitute for a meal.

Four years after Eric's treatments ended, Joan wrote me a letter, once again thanking me for her son's complete recovery. She also told me that Eric has become an outstanding soccer player.

SYMPTOMS OF ALLERGIC REACTIONS TO FOODS

Reports of food allergies began to appear in the medical literature of Europe in the early 1900s, and since the 1940s these allergies have been recognized by doctors around the world. Doctors estimate that more than fifty million people in the United States are affected by food allergies. The symptoms they present with are the following:

- The most common allergic skin reaction to a food is *hives.* Hives are red, very itchy, swollen areas of the skin that may arise suddenly and disappear quickly. They often appear in clusters, with new clusters forming as other areas clear. Hives may occur alone or with other symptoms. Any food can cause hives.
- *Atopic dermatitis,* or *eczema,* a skin condition characterized by itchy, scaly, red skin, can be triggered by a food allergy. This reaction is often chronic, occuring in individuals with personal or family histories of allergies or asthma. Foods high in vitamin C and the B vitamins have been found to be common causes of eczema.
- Symptoms of *asthma,* a chronic disease characterized by attacks in which the airways narrow and the person has difficulty breathing,

may be triggered by a food allergy, especially in infants and children. Foods such as milk, cheese, yeast, sugars, B vitamins, and food additives, including food coloring, are a few examples of the substances that can cause asthma.

- *Gastrointestinal symptoms* of a food allergy can include vomiting, diarrhea, abdominal cramping, sometimes a red rash around the mouth, itching and swelling of the mouth and throat, nausea, abdominal pain, swelling of the stomach, and gas. In infants, *temporary reactions* (not allergies) to certain foods, especially fruits, cow's milk, egg whites, peanuts, and wheat, are common. For example, a rash may appear around the mouth from the natural acids in foods such as tomatoes and oranges. Or an infant may develop diarrhea because of the sugar in fruit juice or another beverage. These symptoms can occur with some frequency, yet still not be classified as allergic reactions. However, other types of reactions *can* be allergic and may be caused by traces of the offending food when eaten again. Colitis can result when yeast, tomatoes, beans, nuts, milk, cheese, sugars, wheat and other grains, fruits, food additives, and toothpaste are ingested by an infant.

- *Headaches or migraines* may be triggered by allergies to foods. Many individuals experience headaches once or twice a day as a reaction to their daily diet. Sugars, eggs, wheat, milk, chocolate, corn, cinnamon, food additives, MSG, and wines are some of the most common offenders.

- *Obesity or weight gain* can be a result of food allergies. Consuming food allergens can trigger the release of insulin, which causes hypoglycemia. This, in turn, may result in uncontrollable hunger, and people may feel a need to eat almost constantly. Frequent overeating causes weight gain. Any food can trigger the symptoms of hypoglycemia, but amino acids, sugars, and carbohydrates such as breads and pasta are the most common offenders.

- *Bad breath* can be caused by allergies to foods. Any food can be the cause, but foods that are difficult for the individual to digest and putrefaction of foods due to maldigestion leads to bad breath.

- *Attention deficit hyperactivity disorder* may be due to food allergies. Sugars, B vitamins, yeast, food additives, milk, corn, and wheat are the most common offenders.
- Confusion, forgetfulness, depression, the inability to concentrate, or other *mental symptoms* may appear within twelve to twenty-four hours of eating a food to which you are allergic. Common foods that can cause these reactions are sugars, carbohydrates, fruits, coffee, and chocolate.
- *Canker sores* and *cold sores* also may be a result of food allergies. Milk, sugars, citrus fruits, and yeast products, as well as the ingredients in toothpaste, are frequent offenders.
- *Recurrent ear infections.* Many children have recurrent ear infections, which begin with an allergic response very similar to the symptoms of an upper respiratory infection. Almost any frequently eaten food can be the culprit, but I have seen milk, sugars, eggs, citrus fruits, fruit juices, wheat, soy, yeast, and corn contribute to the buildup of fluid behind the eardrum, and that fluid predisposes the child to ear infections.
- *Bulimia or other eating disorders.* I see many people, mostly teenage girls and adult women, who have an eating disorder or are recovering from one. They have similar stories and similar food allergies. Food allergies cause cravings. Carbohydrates, chocolate, sugars, and food additives are some of the most common offenders, but any food can be a potential allergen.
- *Arthritic pain, joint pain, and swelling* are often a result of food allergies. The offending foods are commonly sugars, wheat and other grains, acid-producing foods such as red meat, carbohydrates, and members of the nightshade family, including tomatoes, potatoes, green peppers, eggplants, turnips, tobacco, and pimientos.
- *Fatigue* is most often a result of food allergies. Common foods

contributing to fatigue are sugars, coffee, wheat, milk products, fruits, and oats.

- *Premenstrual symptoms and menopausal symptoms* can be related to food allergies. The usual offenders are similar for both syndromes: sugars, citrus, soy, corn, wheat, chocolate, tomatoes, salt, vegetables, and meat.

- *Infertility* can be a result of allergies. The main offender may be food, but there are many other allergens involved in infertility. The foods that cause this condition are carbohydrates, red meat, yeast, milk, fruits, and chicken.

- *Other allergic symptoms* to note include muscle cramping, visual problems, ringing in the ears or earaches, sore throat, hoarseness or cough, nervousness, anxiety, insomnia, night sweats, and hair loss.

It goes without saying that there can be other medical reasons for all of those complaints. But if you have already explored these with your doctor, and she or he cannot explain why you are having these symptoms, then you should consider being tested for food allergies. The list of symptoms above includes only a few of the many possibilities.

✌∅ RONALD'S STORY

Ronald, a twelve-year-old boy, came to my office complaining of migraines and headaches accompanied by dizziness, light-headedness, and night sweats. He was a very active child who played many sports, but his debilitating headaches caused him to miss school and sports practice often. His parents had taken him to many physicians, including chiropractors and psychologists, with only partial success. Nothing seemed really to eliminate his chronic headaches and migraines. The only real help were pain medications, but they also were not preventative. Ronald took ibuprofen daily, and one doctor had recommended Naprosyn, another anti-inflammatory medication. But Ronald's parents had become disillusioned with the recommendations of conventional medicine, which had produced only limited results, and so, on the recommendation of friends, they brought him to my office.

After a taking a thorough history and conducting an examination of Ronald, I made an important discovery. His headaches had been chronic since he was a small child, and manifested after a meal. But his migraines had begun when he entered puberty, about one year before. I began to wonder if an underlying sensitivity to testosterone wasn't a major factor.

After completing Ronald's enzyme and nutritional examination, I explained in detail to him and his parents that he was not properly digesting sugars. I then prescribed to Ron an enzyme to facilitate sugar digestion, and put him on a reduced-carbohydrate diet. During that same visit I performed an allergy test that revealed allergies to eggs, milk, sugars, vitamin C, B vitamins, amino acids, phenolics, yeast, chocolate, spices, beans, corn, turkey, and testosterone. I then began his BioSET™ allergy elimination treatments. After the completion of the sugar treatment, supplemented with digestive enzymes, Ronald noticed that his headaches had begun to diminish and that his energy level had increased. I also treated him for a testosterone allergy, as this hormone is found in many meats, chicken, and other animal products. The treatments were successful—miraculous, as Ron's father said. Ron had no more migraines after those two allergy treatments. I remember his mother commenting, "My son is his old self again. He no longer needs any medication." We did go on and finish clearing the remaining food offenders, although I have seen in my experience that many foods can be cleared simply by treating for phenolics, which are highly allergenic compounds found in many problem foods.

While any system in the body can be affected, most individuals who are sensitive have a target organ that is affected when they encounter any allergy. For some people, the colon may be the most affected, causing bloating and constipation or diarrhea. For others, it may be their stomach, resulting in heartburn, reflux, and nausea.

Foods can be our body's best medicine and true enjoyment for our senses, but foods can also cause infinite havoc in our body-mind. If you have symptoms that occur every day at the same time, whether they are fatigue, a minor headache, or feelings of irritability, they might very well be a result of that well-balanced breakfast you ate. Was it the coffee, the orange juice, the whole-wheat bread, or a combination of all of them? In the rest of this book you will learn what an allergy means for you, how to test for it, and how to rid yourself of your distress. Then your foods really can be delectable.

SELF-ASSESSMENT

The following self-assessment questionnaire will help you determine whether you have the symptoms that commonly indicate food allergies.

CHILDHOOD SYMPTOMS

1. As an infant, did you have any problems tolerating formula or breast milk?
2. Did you have problems with gaining weight, colic, or spitting up during infancy?
3. As an infant, did you suffer from respiratory or skin problems?
4. Were you "difficult" in infancy and/or childhood, often crying or irritable, overactive or underactive? Did you have problems sleeping or trouble learning or paying attention at school?
5. As a child, were you often sick, plagued by ear infections, sore throats, swollen glands, colds, bronchitis, croup, stomachaches, constipation, diarrhea, or headaches?
6. Was your birth difficult or complicated?

PHYSICAL SYMPTOMS

7. As an adult, are you always tired, even though you get enough sleep?
8. Do you frequently have puffy eyes, wrinkles around the eyes, or dark circles under the eyes? Itchy, red, watery, burning, painful, or light-sensitive eyes? Blurred vision? Baggy, swollen eyelids?
9. Do you often have a stuffy, watery, runny nose? Do you sneeze several times in a row? Do you rub your nose upward or wiggle it? Do you have one cold after another without feeling sick? Nosebleeds? Excessive mucus?

10. Do you have asthma or wheezing? Do you cough or wheeze with laughter, with exercise, with cold air, with cold drinks, at night, when it's damp outside?

11. Do you have skin rashes such as eczema or atopic dermatitis? Itchy rashes or hives, especially in your arm or leg creases? Cracked toenails or fingernails? Acne? Dandruff? Hair loss?

12. Do you have recurrent earaches? Fluid behind your eardrums? On-and-off hearing trouble? Ears popping or ringing? Red earlobes? Dizziness? Itchy ears? Drainage from your ear?

13. Do you suffer from digestive problems? Swelling or soreness of your face and lips? Itchy roof of the mouth? Canker sores? Bleeding gums? Bad breath? Nausea and stomachaches? Excess gas, diarrhea, constipation? Belching? Itchy rectal area? Ulcers? Colitis?

14. Do you have difficulty gaining or losing weight? Do you engage in binge eating?

15. Are you a picky eater?

16. Do you have repeated bladder infections, difficulty urinating, or water retention?

17. Is your pulse or heartbeat irregular after eating?

18. Have you ever had seizures?

19. Do you have sinus problems, eye pain, conjunctivitis, sore throat, headaches, dizziness, convulsion, insomnia, leg or muscle aches, back pain, swollen or stiff joints, arthritis, or a constant low-grade fever? Do you feel flushed or chilled, or have excessive sweating or fainting spells?

20. Do you have an unusually pale complexion, or a bloated or puffy face?

21. Do certain foods seem to bring on a headache?

22. Have you been told you have bad breath?

23. Are you or have you ever been bulimic, or experienced any kind of eating disorder?

24. Do you perspire excessively? Do you experience abnormal body odor?

25. Do you experience restless legs? Cramping in your legs and feet?

GENETIC SYMPTOMS

26. Do any blood relatives suffer from allergy syndromes such as hay fever, asthma, skin rashes, or severe reactions to drugs or insect stings?

27. Does anyone in your family have diabetes or low blood sugar, arthritis, headaches, or digestive disorders?

28. Were any blood relatives hyperactive, learning-disabled, or bed-wetters as children?

29. Does anyone in your family suffer from addictive disorders such as alcohol or drug abuse or compulsive eating?

EMOTIONAL SYMPTOMS

30. Did your mother experience severe stress during her pregnancy with you?

31. Do you feel as though you are high one moment and low the next, with bouts of depression appearing for no reason?

32. Do you have trouble concentrating, and sometimes feel confused and spacy?

33. Are you hyperactive, overly nervous, frequently anxious, quick to anger?

34. Does a change in your surroundings or the seasons change how you feel?

If you responded to this questionnaire with a significant number of yes answers, it is likely that you are suffering from food allergies.

During my over twenty years of practice, I have found that there is a profound association between food allergies and many chronic health problems. In fact, I believe food allergies are the root causes of many illnesses physicians encounter in their offices daily.

DEFINING FOOD ALLERGIES

An allergy is an abnormal, adverse physical reaction to certain substances called allergens (or antigens). These substances can be either toxins, such as automobile exhaust fumes or pesticides, or nontoxins, such as pollens or food. Allergy sufferers react to them in small quantities that are harmless to most people.

When exposed to allergens, allergic individuals develop an excess of an antibody called immunoglobulin E (IgE). These IgE antibodies react with allergens to release histamines and other chemicals from cell tissues, producing various allergic symptoms, such as watery eyes and a runny nose. In other words, the immune system mistakenly identifies harmless substances as dangerous invaders and activates an antibody attack to defend the body. The development of an allergy begins when we become sensitized to the substance during our first contact with it, usually without symptoms. Only upon reexposure do the previously created antibodies become active and begin to produce allergy symptoms.

Although a person can develop allergies to practically any substance, the most common allergens include pollen, dust, dust mites, animal dander (from skin, saliva, hair or fur), feathers, cosmetics, mold, insect venom, certain chemicals, drugs (especially penicillin), and foods. We can have an allergic reaction to something after it is inhaled, injected, or ingested or comes in contact with our skin. Allergic reactions can involve any part of the body but most frequently affect the nose, lungs, skin, and eyes.

There are millions of allergy sufferers in the United States—the American Academy of Allergy, Asthma, and Immunology indicates that more than fifty million Americans have allergic diseases. Allergies can emerge at any age without prior warning. Many studies have shown conclusively that parents with allergies will tend to have children with allergies. Some research suggests that the tendency to develop allergies of *some kind* is inherited, but not the tendency to develop a *particular* allergy.

Part of the difficulty in determining how many people actually suffer from allergies lies in how broadly or narrowly one defines the term.

Medical doctors and scientists often hold to a narrow definition, asserting that the only true allergies are those that result from the activation of IgE antibodies. However, millions of people experience allergic symptoms without this IgE antibody reaction. These people can be said to have an intolerance, or hypersensitivity, to particular substances. Although the causes may differ, the diagnosis and treatment of allergy and intolerance often overlap. As a result, allergy research and information do not benefit just those with traditional allergies.

Allergies can cause a predisposition to colds and flu by compromising the immune system and lowering resistance. Once the body becomes host to viruses it can be difficult to distinguish a cold from an allergic reaction, especially since the two will often occur simultaneously. However, allergies do not generally cause fever, and unlike colds, which linger for only a week or two, allergies may refuse to go away.

In this book, I will take a wider view of an allergy, as any negative or abnormal response in the immune system. For example, I believe there is no such thing as a simple cold. A cold is the response of a challenged immune system, whether challenged by a food, a pollen, or a virus. Since a virus is also an allergen in that it stimulates a response by the body, BioSET™ treats a cold like an allergy, with excellent results.

TYPES OF ALLERGIES

Allergies can be classified by either the substance that causes them or the resulting symptoms. Other categories include active or acute allergies and hidden or chronic allergies.

The first category—what causes allergies—includes:

- Ingestants, such as food or food additives
- Inhalants, such as dust
- Contactants, such as latex chemicals or insect bites
- Injectants, such as drugs
- Infectants, such as viruses or bacteria

- Physical agents, such as cold or heat
- Allergies to hormones, such as one's own thyroxine, estrogen, testosterone, or adrenaline
- Allergies of the organs

The category of symptoms caused by allergies includes:

- Hay fever symptoms
- Asthma
- Skin conditions, such as eczema, hives, and rashes
- Headaches and migraines
- Stomach upset
- Chronic fatigue
- Depression
- Chronic pain
- Conjunctivitis
- Anaphylactic shock

Active or acute allergies can be of the immediate type, which means that the symptoms (hives, itching, vomiting, coughing, wheezing, etc.) appear within seconds of every exposure and usually subside within an hour. Or they can be of the delayed type, which means that the reaction occurs hours or days after contact; in such cases the allergen may not be a food itself, but a chemical by-product of the digestion of that particular food.

Hidden allergies may cause chronic developmental and functional problems or severe deficiencies and chemical imbalances. For example, an allergy to B vitamins can cause B vitamin deficiencies and result in health problems such as chronic fatigue, attention deficit hyperactivity disorder, depression, digestive problems, asthma, and headaches. An allergy to calcium can cause joint problems.

FOOD ALLERGIES

A true food allergy is an adverse reaction to a food or food component that involves the body's immune system. Some other adverse reactions to foods might involve the body's metabolism but not the immune system. These reactions are known as food intolerances. Examples of food intolerances are the inability to properly digest certain food components such as lactose (milk sugar). The difference is that a genuine food allergy is caused by antibodies that can be identified by blood testing, while food intolerance is a broader term involving the body's metabolism encompassing many illnesses caused by food. A food intolerance does not register on conventional allergy tests, although it can be measured using bioenergetic testing, such as muscle testing.

A true allergic reaction to a food involves three primary components:

1. Contact with food allergens (the reaction-provoking substance). For example, protein is a common food allergen.
2. Immunoglobulin E (IgE), the antibody in the immune system that reacts with allergens.
3. Mast cells (tissue cells) and basophils (blood cells), which release histamine or other substances causing allergic symptoms when the antigen contacts IgE antibodies on the mast cell.

The body's immune system identifies an allergen in the food as a foreign substance and produces antibodies to halt the "invasion." As the battle rages, symptoms appear throughout the body. The most common sites are the mouth (swelling of the lips), the digestive tract (stomach cramps, vomiting, diarrhea), the skin (hives, rashes, or eczema), the airways (wheezing or breathing problems), the joints (pain), and the head (headaches, migraines). On occasion an allergen will cause a person to go into anaphylaxis, a severe, life-threatening reaction. In extreme cases an individual can have an allergic reaction to minute amounts of the allergen, which might include touching the food with the skin or kissing someone who has eaten the food.

✐ LAURA'S STORY

Laura, a forty-six-year-old woman, came to my office a few months ago. She stated on her history form that she had severe food allergies. We reviewed her history, in which she reported incidents of severe adverse reactions to foods under very extraordinary circumstances. For example, Laura is allergic to peanuts. To show how badly she reacted to them, she shared this story. Once she was in a meeting with an employee who prior to the meeting had eaten some peanuts and failed to wash his hands. He greeted Laura by shaking her hand and speaking to her. During the meeting Laura began to break out in hives and her breathing became restricted. She asked to be immediately escorted to the hospital. The only explanation she could come up with for her reaction was the peanuts she had been exposed to through the handshake and the breath of her colleague. If her colleague had washed his hands and brushed his teeth, she may not have reacted. Laura also told me that she was not able to go to a movie theater due to her allergies to corn and other foods that are often eaten there. She could not be within thirty feet of an allergen, which, of course, made it impossible for her to attend many public events. She was seriously in need of my help.

Almost immediately upon receiving treatment, Laura's reactions lessened and her ability to eat a wider variety of foods increased. Soon after her treatments began, her mother called me and thanked me for the miracles occurring in Laura's life.

Food reactions can be classified as immediate, delayed, or hidden. They may also be thermal, in which symptoms occur after the ingestion of a specific food followed by the subject's exposure to cold, heat, or light.

Children with food allergies experience a wide variety of symptoms, including abdominal pain, headaches, runny noses, asthma, chronic coughing, attention problems, and behavioral problems. Many feel that these allergies disappear as a child matures to adulthood, but in reality they do not. Often some of the acute symptoms lessen over time, but the allergy really becomes chronic or hidden, potentially causing development or functional problems and persistent maladies.

While up to 25 percent of adults believe they have food allergies, conventional Western medicine claims that only 1 percent or 2 percent actually do. Those who do not have allergies according to the strict definition have what traditional doctors usually call a food intolerance. Some causes of food intolerances are chemicals, such as caffeine, and food colorings, such as tartrazine, which do not produce adverse effects in the majority of the population but do trigger allergic symptoms in some people. Of course, to those who have them, these food intolerances can be equally uncomfortable. A deficiency of enzymes (the chemicals that help digestion) can cause problems as well. If a person lacks one or more enzymes, she may experience digestive problems such as diarrhea and stomach pain after consuming foods the missing enzymes would normally digest. For example, people who have difficulty drinking milk are unable to produce lactase, the enzyme that digests lactose, the sugar in milk. In my clinical practice I have found that most lactose-intolerant people who are treated for this condition with the BioSET™ allergy elimination technique are then fully able to tolerate milk, with no side effects.

Finally, studies indicate that taking antibiotics can increase the chances of food intolerance in some people. Antibiotics apparently kill some types of bacteria in the large intestine and allow others to flourish, causing an abnormal reaction during digestion that produces various unpleasant by-products and associated symptoms. Antibiotics can also cause candida (yeast) overgrowth in the intestines, which can lead to an imbalance with healthy intestinal flora or microorganisms. I have had successful results in treating candida and other pathogens with the BioSET™ system.

LIFE-THREATENING REACTIONS

A small percentage of food-allergic individuals have severe reactions, called anaphylaxis. Anaphylaxis is a rare but potentially fatal condition in which several different parts of the body experience allergic reactions simultaneously, causing hives, swelling of the throat, and difficulty breathing.

Symptoms usually appear rapidly, sometimes within minutes of exposure to the allergen. Because they can be life-threatening, immediate medical attention is necessary when an anaphylactic reaction occurs. Standard emergency treatment often includes an injection of epinephrine (adrenaline) to open up the airway and blood vessels.

CATEGORIES OF FOOD ALLERGENS

Food allergens are those parts of foods that cause allergic reactions. All foods can cause reactions, but some are more potent allergens than others. The most common food allergens—responsible for up to 90 percent of all allergic reactions—are the proteins in cow's milk, eggs, peanuts, wheat, soy, fish, shellfish, and tree nuts. Protein foods tend to be more allergenic than other foods, since proteins can be more difficult to digest than fats and carbohydrates. When the digestion of proteins is not complete, the undigested molecules are absorbed into the bloodstream. The immune system then interprets these unprocessed food molecules as foreign substances rather than as nutrients, and an allergic response occurs. Also, when there is an inadequate breakdown of the amino acids within protein, a deficiency can result despite sufficient levels of high-quality protein in the diet. The consequences of this deficiency may be an inability to produce adequate levels of enzymes, hormones, antibodies, and immune factors. This can then create a vicious circle, because adequate enzymes are not available to digest the next ingested protein.

All foods come from either a plant or an animal source, and foods are grouped into families according to their origin. Peanuts, black-eyed peas, kidney beans, lima beans, and soybeans are members of the legume family, whereas asparagus, chives, garlic, and onion are—perhaps surprisingly—members of the lily family. In some food groups, especially tree nuts and seafood, an allergy to one member of the food family may result in the person being allergic to all the members of the same group. This is known as *cross reactivity.*

Cross reactivity between foods and pollens heightens symptoms for some people. Bananas, watermelon, zucchini, honeydew, cucumbers, and other members of the gourd family cross-react with ragweed pollen, which means that their allergy-producing proteins are identical. As a result, a person sensitive to ragweed could react with symptoms the first time he or she consumes watermelon, a cucumber, or a banana. Birch pollen cross-reacts with potatoes, carrots, celery, hazelnuts, and apples.

Within animal groups of foods, cross reactivity is not as common. For example, people allergic to cow's milk can usually eat beef, and patients allergic to eggs can usually eat chicken. People allergic to eggs usually react only to the egg white, which contains several proteins. However, because it is impossible to completely avoid cross-contamination between yolk and white, they must avoid eggs completely.

Some people may be allergic to both peanuts and walnuts, which are actually from different food families. These kinds of allergies are called *coincidental allergies* because they are really not related, even though they might seem to be.

A *concomitant allergy* is one that causes reactions when another allergen, such as a chemical or a particulate inhalant (pollen, dust, or mold), is present. For example, if wheat or a product containing wheat is eaten while ragweed is pollinating, one may experience an allergic reaction. Reactions to a concomitant food can occur up to six weeks after the pollen season is over.

Here is a list of some plants and their related food allergies.

SUBSTANCE	ASSOCIATED FOODS
GRASSES	Legumes: beans, peas, soybeans, cottonseed oil
	Grains: wheat, corn, rye, barley, oats, rice, mullet
TREES	
Cedar, juniper	Beef, yeast (baker's, brewer's), malt
Cottonwood	Lettuce
Elm	Milk, mint
Oak	Eggs, apples
Pecan, hickory	Corn, bananas
Mesquite	Cane sugar, oranges

SUBSTANCE	ASSOCIATED FOODS
WEEDS	
Ragweed, short and western	Egg
Ragweed, giant	Milk, mint
Sage	Potatoes, tomatoes
Amaranth family (pigweed, carelessweed)	Pork, black pepper
Marsh elder	Wheat
DUST	Oysters, clams, scallops

TYPES OF ALLERGIC REACTIONS

A synergistic allergy, or combination reaction, occurs when someone eats two or more foods that do not provoke any reaction when eaten by themselves. For example, a person may experience an allergic reaction when she eats corn and any vegetable oil at the same meal, but not when she eats corn or vegetable oil alone. Synergistic allergies are actually very common. Some recognized synergistic foods are cane sugar and oranges, corn and bananas, milk and mint, eggs and apples, pork and black pepper, and beef and yeast (baker's, brewer's, malt). Other possible synergistic foods are wheat and tea, milk and chocolate, pork and chicken, cola and chocolate, coffee and cola, and coffee and chocolate.

Food allergies can be harder to recognize than other allergies, such as airborne substances, because food allergies might not be felt until the food is broken down by digestion. For some people who eat a food to which they are allergic, their lips, mouth, and throat begin to swell or itch even before the food reaches their stomach. But many people feel their symptoms after the food is digested, resulting in anything from nausea and queasiness to gas, bloating, diarrhea, headaches, depression, and brain fog. These symptoms can take hours or days to appear. I have seen an allergy to a food affect someone up to ten days after eating it; in this case, it was an oatmeal cookie, to which the individual was highly allergic, and it took another ten days for her symptoms to finally disappear.

Food allergies sometimes don't occur every time you eat that food. The frequency of the reaction is determined by the severity of the food allergy, a response that I am able to test. Some foods will always produce allergic reactions, but other, more mildly allergenic foods do not always produce reactions. As noted previously, I have named this the *load phenomenon*.

In my estimation, over 90 percent of the population has either food allergies or food intolerances, most of which are genetic in origin. However, in the majority of people these allergies are hidden or inactive. It is the load phenomenon that activates these allergies in certain people. If over a period of time someone with a hidden allergy confronts other, more active or acute allergens, or if she is physically, mentally, or emotionally stressed—for example, she lacks sufficient sleep or eats poorly—the hidden allergy may become pronounced. The body falls prey to other problems as its resistance breaks down, and for the first time one may experience allergy-related symptoms such as asthma, arthritis, swelling, chronic pain, headaches, or chronic fatigue.

ᗯᗣ JANET'S STORY

I saw the load phenomenon at work with Janet, a fifty-three-year-old woman who came into my office complaining of asthma and chronic sinusitis. Janet had previously experienced a stuffy nose from time to time, but she had never been asthmatic. About two years before, when the asthma began, she had a bad case of flu that kept her home from work for a month. Around the same time she was experiencing other serious stresses, her mother died of cancer, and Janet began to notice premenopausal symptoms. After a thorough examination, I began some allergy testing. I found Janet to be very allergic to hormones, flu viruses, certain environmental and chemical substances, sugar, dairy products, grains, and many other foods. She was particularly intolerant of sugars and carbohydrates and was unable to absorb these foods.

It soon became apparent to me that Janet was experiencing the allergic load phenomenon. She was living on pasta and bread, foods she did not digest well, and she had never fully recovered from the flu virus, which I also considered an allergic reaction. The death of her mother had added to her stress, and her premenopausal state had caused hormonal fluctuations and further stress. With her immune system compromised, certain hidden allergies began to manifest themselves. Janet became overly sensitive to foods she had never noticed reactions to before, such as corn, honey, and cheese, and these provoked her asthma attacks. Although this extreme response didn't develop overnight, I believe most of Janet's food allergies were there from the beginning.

Mild food allergies can be tolerated if you eat only a small amount of that food. Sometimes, with certain allergies, cooking breaks down food to a degree that makes it possible to eat it without serious reactions. For example, one may discover that eating tomatoes raw produces a severe reaction, but that cooked tomatoes do not cause such a problem. This is often the case with foods such as tomatoes, celery, and snap peas.

An interesting observation I have made is that allergic reactions to foods are not always uncomfortable. In fact, you may feel better after eating certain allergenic foods. Doctors call this reaction *allergic addiction* and compare it to the temporary lift many smokers feel after a cigarette. This lift often creates a food craving, which may very well point to a food to which you are highly allergic.

My belief is that the craving for or addiction to a particular food is caused by one of the substances in that food. If someone has a fundamental allergy to a substance and therefore cannot utilize it properly in the body, a deficiency in that substance can result. Therefore the craving for the food is actually a craving to fulfill that deficiency. For example, many people are allergic to vitamin C. Vitamin C, as we all know, has a wide range of applications in the treatment and prevention of many diseases. It is vital in combating disease, healing muscle tissue, and helping to protect the bronchial airways and lungs. Vitamin C is a primary antioxidant vitamin, preventing tissue damage and helping white blood cells to fight infections. An allergy to vitamin C will cause a craving for foods high in vitamin C, such as oranges, tomatoes, broccoli, strawberries, peppers, and potatoes. Unfortunately, eating these foods does not satisfy the craving if you are allergic to vitamin C. The craving will continue, and ingesting foods containing this vitamin may produce symptoms such as eczema and a chronic sore throat.

DIAGNOSING FOOD ALLERGIES

There are many warning signs that indicate the presence of a food allergy. You can suspect a hidden food allergy when you or your child develops dark circles under the eyes; when you sniff, snort, or clear your throat often, or rub your nose; and when you are nervous, irritable, or overactive, or tired, droopy, or drowsy. Other signs of hidden allergies include headaches, stomachaches, or muscle aches; coughing or wheezing; or irritability and frequent digestive and respiratory problems. One should suspect the presence of hidden allergies when other members of the family are bothered by allergies.

Diagnosing food allergies usually begins with a thorough medical history, a complete physical examination, and selected tests to rule out underlying medical conditions not related to food allergy.

To completely unravel a food allergy problem, you must sort out not only your symptoms but also what you are really eating. Labels on food items do not fully reveal all the ingredients. Some lists of ingredients will just say "vegetable oil," with no description of whether it is corn, safflower, soybean, peanut, olive, or cottonseed oil. Nondairy foods can actually include whey, casein, or lactose under those names or ingredients such as butter, cream, butterfat, whipped cream, skim milk, powdered milk, milk solids, yogurt, sodium or calcium caseinate, sodium or calcium lactate, or lactalbumin. And manufacturers of mayonnaise and ice cream are not obliged to list any ingredients at all.

Eating out in a restaurant can be formidable for allergic individuals. You might think you are eating foods with ingredients that seem straightforward enough. Yet a simple hamburger can contain a dozen other ingredients to which you may be allergic, such as butter, milk, eggs, wheat, rye, black pepper, sugar, vinegar, tomatoes, corn sweetener, and other spices and flavorings.

A food diary can be an invaluable tool in the discovery of food allergies. A record of what you ate, when you ate it, and how you felt immediately after eating it or throughout the day can help identify foods to which you are allergic. It is wise to list all the ingredients of the food in your diary as well as the food itself. Don't rely on your memory. Carefully list each food and all of its ingredients directly after having eaten your meal. Carry the diary with you in your purse or pocket, or use your Palm Pilot or other electronic device. Be sure to include the severity of your symptoms so that you are able to distinguish between mild and severe allergic reactions. It is also advisable to weigh yourself every morning after going to the bathroom, as a sudden weight gain accompanied by increased thirst can indicate fluid retention, which is a symptom of an allergy; noticing that your rings or shoes are tighter is another indicator. Also include frequent urination, urinary urgency, or (for children) bed-wetting.

Selective elimination diets are another tool to evaluate your food intolerances. First, avoid a prime suspect, such as milk or wheat, in all forms. Record how you feel and any lessening of symptoms in your food diary. After a three-week period, eat the food again, preferably in generous portions at several meals, and continue to observe your symptoms. If you experience symptoms, then you are probably allergic to the food.

Obviously, you need to test only the food or foods of which you are unsure. If you suffer anaphylaxis with a certain food, then there is certainly no need to test it. Just avoid it. Selective elimination diets are designed to help people confirm suspicions about a particular food. And they can provide a starting point for those individuals who experience symptoms every day but don't have a clue which foods are to blame. In those cases, you can begin by testing the most common food allergens, such as milk, eggs, wheat, corn, yeast, and beef, to identify some of the main culprits.

The muscle-testing procedure for evaluating food allergies can be made much easier by utilizing this selective elimination regimen. It gives you a place to begin in your testing process. Once you have some idea

SAMPLE OF FOOD DIARY

	Symptoms	Cravings
Upon Arising		
After Breakfast		
After Lunch		
After Supper		
During the Night		
Any drugs that were taken during the day to combat food reactions		

What you ate today/supplements and vitamins

Breakfast	Morning	Lunch	Afternoon	Supper	Evening

about your main allergens, you can do some muscle testing on others that are also suspicious and go on from there until you have determined most of your food allergies.

Rotation diets have been used for many years as a tool to assess food allergies and, even more important, to eliminate them. This type of diet consists of rotating the offending foods every four or five days. First, you should avoid your suspected problem foods completely for up to six months, to give your body a period during which it can rest from its allergies. Then you reintroduce the food to your diet, but no more often than once every four or five days. This rotation allows your antibody levels to subside before you once again consume the food in question. So if you eat eggs on Monday, you shouldn't eat eggs again until Friday or later. A rotation diet increases your tolerance to the food simply by exposing you to it less often.

Rotation diets can be helpful for some, but there are quite a few difficulties. First and most important, many people are allergic not to a food itself but to the substances or compounds found in it, such as phenolics, vitamin C, or selenium. Therefore, avoiding a certain food does not prevent reactions to other foods containing the offending ingredient. Coumarin, a phenolic found in 80 percent of our commonly eaten foods, including dairy products and wheat, is highly allergenic. How can anyone possibly avoid all these foods?

Second, people do not find it easy to follow a rotation diet. When people miss their favorite foods or begin craving the foods to which they are most allergic, they are often unable to refrain from eating them.

Third, you need also to learn about food families. If you are allergic to one food, you should avoid foods from the same family because they can also cause a reaction. For example, asparagus is related to onions and garlic, cucumbers to melons, and carrots to celery. Here are some other food families:

- Cashew   Mango, pistachio
- Apple   Crabapple, pear, quince
- Chocolate   Cocoa, cola, karaya gum
- Mint   Basil, catnip, horehound, lemon balm, marjoram, oregano, rosemary, sage, thyme
- Walnut   Butternut, English walnut, pecan, hickory nut
- Yam   Chinese potato
- Bass   White perch, yellow bass
- Codfish   Cod (scrod), haddock, pollack, whiting
- Flounder   Halibut, sole
- Mackerel   Albacore, bonito, tuna
- Yellow perch Walleye

- Salmon   Salmon, trout
- Clam   Quahog
- Lobster   Crayfish, Langostino
- Shrimp   Prawn

Although the rotation diet has some drawbacks, it can be useful, especially for highly sensitive individuals. Also, cultivating diversity in your diet makes your menus more interesting and helps prevent allergies. There is some evidence that you can actually create a food allergy when you eat the same foods over and over again.

THE HIDDEN ALLERGIES CAUSED BY
BIOTECHNOLOGY OR GENETIC ENGINEERING

Biotechnology uses sophisticated techniques to confer selected characteristics on plants and animals used for food. It is also used to increase agricultural productivity. The great promise behind biotechnology is that the use of these techniques will help solve world food problems by creating a more abundant, more nutritious, and less expensive food supply. Despite this promise, public concern about the safety, usefulness, and social consequences of genetically engineered food products has led to boycotts, legislative bans, and demands for stronger federal regulation. Such actions have caused leaders of the biotechnology industry to identify public "biotechnophobia" as the most serious threat to the commercialization of their products, and to view as their greatest challenge the need to reassure people that these new techniques are both safe and beneficial.

Questions of safety vex federal regulators and industry scientists as well as the public. The transfer of genes from one microbe, plant, or animal into another raises many issues about the unintended consequences of such manipulations. Hidden food allergies could be one such consequence. Genes encode proteins, and proteins can be allergenic. In other words, biotechnology companies might be introducing allergenic proteins from donor organisms into the food supply.

The Food and Drug Administration (FDA) anticipated this problem in 1992 when it devised its policy on transgenic plant foods. But this policy only requires premarketing notification of the FDA, premarketing safety testing, and labeling of food products made with ingredients that include these transferred genes from a small group of the most commonly allergenic foods. For this reason, public-interest groups have cautioned that the existing rules inadequately protect people against lesser-known transgenic allergens to which they might be sensitive.

Food allergens can indeed be transferred from one plant to another by transgenic manipulation—for example, from Brazil nuts to soybeans. As an example, let's take a person who is allergic to the protein that is the principal allergen in the Brazil nut. When she undergoes a standard skin-prick test with extracts of genetically engineered soybeans that contain this protein, she will have a similar allergic response, even though she is not normally allergic to soybeans. Eating genetically engineered soybeans may be quite dangerous for her because nuts are known to cause allergic reactions that range from mild itching to anaphylaxis and sudden death.

Another problem is that most biotechnology companies use microorganisms rather than food plants as gene donors, even though the allergenic potential of these newly introduced microbial proteins is uncertain, unpredictable, and as yet untestable.

Pioneer Hi-Bred International developed transgenic soybeans in an attempt to increase the amount of sulfur-containing amino acids—methionine and cystine—in soy-based animal feeds. Such feeds must otherwise be supplemented with methionine (which can be converted to cystine) to promote optimal growth. The Brazil nut is exceptionally rich in methionine and cystine, so its gene was a logical choice as a donor. Even though Pioneer Hi-Bred developed its soybeans for use in animal feeds, there is no easy method of separating soybeans destined for animals from those slated for human consumption. Soy proteins, which are less allergenic than milk proteins, are used in infant formulas, meat extenders, baked goods, and dairy substitutes. Because the consumption of soy-based foods appears to reduce the risks of heart disease and cancer, the prevalence of soy proteins in foods consumed by infants and adults is sure to increase.

From the standpoint of *human* nutrition, soybeans are just fine the way they are. Their methionine content is sufficient. Even if used as the sole source of dietary protein, soy foods maintain nitrogen balance and support growth in adults, children, and full-term infants. They must be supplemented only when used in feeding premature infants.

The FDA is not required to label most bioengineered foods as such, and this causes serious problems for those with food allergies. This FDA policy would appear to favor industry over consumer protection. Although the labeling of transgenic foods raises complex regulatory issues, surveys indicate strong public support for doing so. The FDA has recently drafted a premarketing notification rule that would require companies to inform the agency when they are developing transgenic foods, in part to help resolve the safety issues related to allergenicity. In the current climate of deregulation, the implementation of any new premarketing notification rule seems unlikely, particularly since the biotechnology industry is demanding that such a requirement be limited in scope and end after three years. The unresolved status of this regulatory policy means that the responsibility for protecting the public against uncommon or unknown allergens in transgenic foods will continue to be delegated to industry and be largely voluntary.

This situation illustrates the pressing need to expand basic and clinical research on food allergies. More information about incidence, prevalence, dietary exposure, immune responses, diagnosis, and treatment would help researchers, regulators, and biotechnology companies predict whether transgenic proteins are likely to cause harm. In the special case of transgenic soybeans, the donor species was known to be allergenic, serum samples from persons allergic to the donor species were available for testing, and the product was withdrawn. The next case could be less ideal and the public less fortunate. It is in everyone's best interest to develop regulatory policies for transgenic foods that include premarketing notification and labeling.

Industry benefits when the public is convinced that transgenic foods are safe, and stronger federal regulations would encourage such public confidence.

FOOD ADDITIVES AND FOOD LABELING

Food additives can be a huge offender for the food allergy sufferer. If you are not allergic to the food itself, you may be allergic to a food coloring, preservative, or other additive. For example, additives such as MSG, a common flavor enhancer, and BHT and BHA, which are preservatives, can cause a serious reaction in asthmatics. Food dyes such as tartrazine, which is found in FD&C Yellow No. 5, the most common artificial food coloring, can cause hives, hyperactivity, behavioral problems, and eczema, as can other food additives such as sodium benzoate and sulfur dioxide.

Many food additives and artificial colors are made from coal tar or petroleum. Many fruits such as oranges, bananas, pears, peaches, and tomatoes are picked before they are ripe and gassed with ethylene, a petroleum-based chemical that hastens ripening. If you are allergic to petroleum in the air, you are likely going to react to the foods containing this chemical.

Food labeling is much less complete than allergy sufferers and BioSET™ practitioners would like. The biggest problem is that many foods are exempt from listing ingredients on their labels. These rules behind food labeling are called the Standards of Identity. The Standards of Identity were established years ago by the FDA and require foods such as bread, catsup, and mayonnaise to contain certain standard ingredients. For example, a condiment such as mayonnaise must contain eggs, vegetable oil, and vinegar, but none of these ingredients has to be listed.

And this is where those with food allergies can run into a problem. The vegetable oil can be a number of different oils. I have many patients who are allergic to soy, and soy oil is one of the vegetable oils used in some kinds of mayonnaise. The lack of proper labeling can be a nightmare for many. Other problems that can arise are that some kinds of mayonnaise may also contain food additives, food coloring, artificial sweeteners, as well as other highly allergic ingredients. Unfortunately, the Standards of Identity are an imperfect tool.

There are other loopholes in this labeling process. The FDA requires that all ingredients appear on the label in descending order by weight. Specific food additives must be listed, but not specific food colorings and artificial flavors. These can be listed solely as "artificial colors and flavors" without naming the exact substances. Many highly processed foods are guilty of harboring such "hidden" ingredients. Some of these, including FD&C Yellow No. 5 and FD&C Red No. 40 or No. 3, can be possibly fatal for allergy sufferers. Asthmatics can also be very allergic to food colorings. Children with attention deficit hyperactivity disorder are often highly allergic to food coloring and preservatives, so reading food labels is imperative in working with these children. Many allergy sufferers are allergic to natural flavorings, such as strawberry, mint, cinnamon, vanilla, and chocolate. And I have seen patients react from supposedly safe packaged foods sold in health food stores or organic markets.

Metabisulfite and other sulfur-based additives are highly allergenic, especially to asthmatics. These additives are used to preserve many foods and beverages. Most dried foods are treated with sulfur, and so is molasses. Many foods that contain sulfur additives are not labeled as such. Wines are frequently infused with sulfites, but wines and other alcoholic beverages are not required to have their ingredients listed on their labels. Supermarkets have been known to spray metabisulfite or sodium bisulfite on fruit and vegetables to keep them attractive-looking. Fish may be dipped in a solution of metabisulfite to keep it looking fresh. Many salad bars use metabisulfites to keep the lettuce and other raw vegetables from browning. MSG (monosodium glutamate) is the most well known of all the food additives. Common symptoms after eating foods flavored with MSG include migraines, numbness, nausea, dizziness, difficulty breathing, and hives.

Some manufacturers list specific colorings and other additives because of public pressure, but not enough do this. The inadequacy of food labeling is a problem we all face, and until labels are required to list every single ingredient, we must be extra cautious. Allergic individuals should avoid any foods that have the word *artificial* anywhere on the label.

ALLERGIES TO PESTICIDES AND WATER

Allergies to pesticides can complicate the food allergy equation. Foods that normally do not produce a reaction can do so if they are overly laden with pesticides. A person may eat grapes one day and have no allergic reaction. The next time she may react with an asthma attack because the grapes have been sprayed with fumigants (mold inhibitors), herbicides (weed killers), or pesticides (insect and rodent killers). Tree fruits, and in particular peaches, apples, and cherries, are sprayed more often than any crop in the United States. But, unfortunately, no crop goes untouched if that crop was in the vicinity of the spraying, and washing foods often will not get rid of these chemicals. Eating only organically grown food is the ideal we should strive for. I highly recommend organic foods to allergic individuals, especially if you are already aware that you have chemical and environmental sensitivities.

Every so often I will find individuals who are allergic to their water. They exhibit specific allergic reactions when they drink it: hay fever, bronchitis, mouth sores, diarrhea, bloating, urinary incontinence, irritability, anxiety, headaches, and spaciness. Tap water can contain chemicals such as chlorine, fluoride, and formaldehyde, and hormones such as estrogen and testosterone. Although tap water is the kind of water people are most likely to be allergic to, I have seen some people react just as badly to bottled water. The minerals in the water or the plastic in which it is contained can be the culprit.

The muscle-testing procedure is an excellent tool to evaluate your sensitivity to many different waters. Distilled water (water that is heated, turned to steam, and recondensed back to water) is an alternative for highly allergic individuals. In fact, many of my patients decide to use distilled water as their first choice in order to avoid any reactions. But some distilled water can still have remnants of chemicals such as chlorine in it, which can cause reactions in certain highly sensitive individuals. Again, muscle testing is the most reliable way to determine your sensitivity. A water allergy can be treated with the BioSET™ allergy elimination technique.

3

Underlying Components of Food Allergies

If you could listen in on various friends' conversations throughout the day, you would very often hear them talking about foods and their various idiosyncratic experiences after eating them. They might complain about feeling tired, bloated, or irritable; or about having headache pain, swollen legs or fingers, and hives; and, of course, about their continual weight gain. Or they might describe those nasty, undeniable yearnings they have for chocolate or sugar.

For example, two weeks ago I was attending a class with a group of doctors. After lunch, four doctors remarked about how they felt. One doctor had an upset stomach, another felt extremely tired, one complained of a scratchy sore throat, and another noticed an intensification of the ear pain he had been experiencing all week.

This phenomenon occurs with all of us. We are subjected to countless maladies on a daily basis because of those ubiquitous food allergies. We love those foods, we crave those foods, and *we live for those foods.* But are they causing us to feel ill? This chapter unveils the truth behind food allergies, explaining why they play havoc with our bodies and our minds. I will begin by identifying common allergenic foods and the specific ingredients in them that provoke an allergic response.

FOOD INGREDIENTS THAT CAN CAUSE ALLERGIES

The specific foods themselves are not always the culprit in the allergic response; frequently it is one or more of the substances that make up those foods. It might surprise you to learn that the most common problematic substances are the vitamins and minerals inherent in foods (see Appendix 3). They can cause us to have allergic reactions to many foods we eat on a daily basis.

ALLERGIES TO CALCIUM

The first such substance is calcium, a mineral essential for the maintenance of the body's bones and nervous system. Milk, dairy products, and root and green vegetables are all high in calcium, as are sesame seeds, oats, navy beans, dry beans, almonds, walnuts, peanuts, sunflower seeds, sardines, and salmon. When individuals are allergic to calcium, they may have difficulty absorbing and utilizing it. This can then cause symptoms of calcium deficiency, such as joint pain or aches, crackling noises in joints, osteoporosis, menstrual leg cramps, tetany, headache, hyperactivity, restlessness (calcium is essential for relaxation and sleep), abdominal pain, skin problems, canker sores, recurrences of herpes, obesity, arthritis pain, or insomnia.

A three-year-old boy named Jason came to see me at my clinic many years ago. Jason had difficulty sleeping at night, and his mother suspected this problem might be due to environmental allergies. After I treated Jason for calcium with BioSET™, he never experienced problems with sleeping again.

VITAMIN C ALLERGIES

Vitamin C, which is taken as a supplement by many people, is another common allergen. You may wonder how anyone could be allergic to such an essential vitamin, but plenty of individuals are. Vitamin C is found in fresh fruits and vegetables, including rose hips, citrus fruits, black currants, apples, strawberries, guavas, cherries, potatoes, cabbage, broccoli, tomatoes, turnip greens, bell peppers, green and leafy vegetables, cauliflower, and sweet potatoes. Many people do not realize that foods are the best source of vitamin C, not the high-dosage supplements that many people take. When a vitamin C allergy is cleared, allergies to many fruits and vegetables are automatically cleared.

Everyone knows that scurvy is caused by a vitamin C deficiency. But most people don't realize that fatigue is a symptom of scurvy. As in the case of calcium, a vitamin C allergy can cause a deficiency in this vitamin because the body cannot digest it. This results in tiredness, lethargy, and exhaustion. Other common allergic symptoms associated with a vitamin C allergy are chronic sore throats and eczema. In fact, it is very common for eczema sufferers to have an allergy to vitamin C and foods containing high amounts of vitamin C. I have treated many individuals who suffer from frequent colds and flu due to an allergy to vitamin C and their body's inability to use it properly.

Leslie, a twenty-five-year-old asthmatic referred to me by another health practitioner, had been prescribed high doses of vitamin C for her severe wheezing and restricted breathing. This is a common therapeutic regimen for asthma sufferers.

But this patient noticed that not only had the vitamin C failed to help her, she began to experience overwhelming fatigue, joint and kidney pain, headaches, and indigestion when she began to take the supplements.

When I tested her, I found that she was allergic to vitamin C. After I treated her for this allergy with the BioSET™ allergy elimination technique, I recommended that she continue with the vitamin C dosage prescribed by her other practitioner. Once her allergy was cleared, she greatly benefited from her vitamin C supplementation and her asthma improved tremendously.

ALLERGIES TO B VITAMINS

Another significant vitamin allergy that we need to be aware of is an allergy to B vitamins. This allergy is extremely critical because the B vitamins are found in virtually every food. The only foods I have found that do not contain them are tapioca, Jell-O, and Cool Whip—not exactly a healthy diet.

There are eleven different B vitamins. They are: B_1, thiamin; B_2, riboflavin; B_3, niacin or nicotinic acid; B_5, pantothenic acid; B_6, pyridoxine; B_{12}, cobalamin; vitamin H; biotin; choline; inositol; PABA; and folic acid.

B vitamins are essential for the emotional, physical, and psychological well-being of the body. They contribute to maintaining a healthy nervous system and aid in the digestion of fats and protein. People allergic to B vitamins may suffer severe depression, cloudy thinking, exhaustion, mood swings, and nervousness, and may react adversely to almost every food they eat.

B vitamins are also used therapeutically for the treatment of skin disorders and respiratory problems, and can help to prevent colds and improve memory. Inositol, biotin, and choline prevent hair loss and are essential for healthy hair. Folic acid is needed for the formation of red blood cells and the prevention of a certain type of anemia. Obviously, allergies to the B vitamins must be cleared if good health is to be maintained.

Joan, age thirty-six, came to see me with severe depression. Her condition had become critical, and she was taking large doses of several medications. I began to treat her with the BioSET™ allergy elimination technique. After I had desensitized her to vitamin C and the B vitamins, I prescribed an enzyme formulation that included these vitamins, allowing for their optimal absorption. Overnight her depression improved dramatically, and she was able to reduce her medications.

For most people who suffer from a chronic health problem, whether it is fatigue, eczema, depression, or arthritis, a B vitamin allergy may be a factor. Clearing the B vitamins may also clear allergies to other substances high in B vitamins, such as wheat and many other grains, some vegetables, potatoes, brewer's yeast, and meat. Whole-grain allergies seem to be the most positively affected by clearing allergies to the B vitamins. People who crave carbohydrates usually have a B vitamin allergy.

The B vitamins are synergistic, which means that they work as a team to perform all their vital individual functions properly and are more potent when taken together than separately. Hence, many nutritionists recommend taking a B vitamin complex rather than single vitamins. For proper metabolism of the B vitamins, the body must also maintain adequate levels of other nutrients such as iron and enzymes. Thiamin, riboflavin, and niacin all bind to enzymes to help them do their job.

The primary function of B vitamins is to convert carbohydrates, fats, and proteins into energy the body can use. They are also vital to the proper functioning of the nervous system, the production of red blood cells, the maintenance of muscle tone in the gastrointestinal tract, and the health of the skin, hair, eyes, mouth, and liver. A high-potency vitamin B complex can be useful in recovering from debilitating illness, alcoholism, or excessive medication use because it helps reduce the effects of stress and supports the adrenal glands. Supplementation with B vitamins is recommended for heavy coffee drinkers, women who take birth control pills, and people with high-sugar diets.

B_1, or thiamin, aids in the digestion of carbohydrates, stabilizes the appetite, promotes growth and good muscle tone, inhibits pain, and assists in the normal functioning of the nervous system, muscles, and heart. Thiamin helps the body to release energy from carbohydrates during metabolism. People who expend more energy and have a high caloric intake need more thiamin than those who eat fewer calories. This vitamin can be depleted by excessive consumption of alcoholic beverages. A person deficient in B_1 might experience loss of appetite and weight, feelings of weakness and tiredness, paralysis, nervousness, irritability, insomnia, unfamiliar aches and pains, depression, heart difficulties, or constipation and gastrointestinal problems. A thiamin deficiency can also cause the disease beriberi, which results in weakness, nervous tingling, and poor coordination.

Grain products, including bread, cereals, pasta, and rice, are good sources of thiamin. Others sources are meat (especially pork), poultry, and fish; fruits and vegetables; and sunflower seeds. Pasta, most instant and ready-to-eat cereals, and most breads made from refined flour are enriched with vitamins, including thiamin, to replace the nutrients lost in processing.

Vitamin B_2, or riboflavin, is necessary for the metabolism of carbohydrates, fats, and protein. B_2 also promotes general health by maintaining cell respiration, aiding in the formation of antibodies and red blood cells, ensuring good vision, relieving eye fatigue, and maintaining healthy nails and hair. The body's need for riboflavin may increase during periods of healing and pregnancy and in conditions such as asthma. A person deficient in B_2 might experience sluggishness; itchy, burning, or bloodshot eyes; sores or cracks in and around the mouth and lips, or a purplish or inflamed tongue and mouth; dermatitis; oily skin; slowed growth; trembling; digestive problems; and respiratory problems.

Breads, cereals and other grain products, milk and milk products, meat, poultry, and fish are all good sources of riboflavin. Pasta and most breads made from refined flours are enriched with riboflavin, since riboflavin is another of the nutrients lost in processing. To retain riboflavin during storage, food should be stored in containers that light cannot pass through. Vegetables should be cooked in minimal amounts of water to retain this vitamin, and meat should be roasted or broiled.

Vitamin B_3, also called niacin or niacinamide, helps to improve circulation and reduce the blood's cholesterol level. B_3 also assists in maintaining the nervous system and cell respiration. It aids in metabolizing protein, sugar, and fat; helps to reduce high blood pressure; increases energy through the proper use of food; produces acid; metabolizes sex hormones; activates histamines; and prevents pellagra (a deficiency disease characterized by diarrhea and dermatitis). It also helps to maintain healthy skin, tongue, and digestion. The body requires more niacin during periods of stress, acute illness, and low intake of tryptophan, an essential amino acid found in meat, poultry, fish, and eggs.

B_3, niacin, is a good example of how a vitamin can be as effective as drugs in combating disease. Niacin, which is much less expensive than prescription medication, is successfully being used to lower levels of harmful cholesterol (LDL) and raise levels of good cholesterol (HDL).

A person deficient in B_3 might experience gastrointestinal disturbances, loss of appetite, indigestion, bad breath, canker sores, skin disorders or rashes, muscular weakness, fatigue, insomnia, vague aches and pains, headaches, nervousness, memory loss, irritability, or depression. A lack of this vitamin might also result in respiratory problems (including asthma and chronic bronchitis) or pellagra.

Niacin can be formed in the body from tryptophan, an essential amino acid found in meat, poultry, fish, and eggs. If your diet includes these foods, you will have less need to supplement niacin from other sources. Other good sources of B_3 itself are meat, poultry, fish (especially tuna), bread, cereals, other grain products such as wheat bran, vegetables such as mushrooms and asparagus, and peanuts. Pasta and breads made from refined flours are usually fortified with niacin. Loss of niacin from foods due to preparation and storage is slight, but vegetables should be cooked in a minimal amount of water, and meat should be roasted or broiled to retain this nutrient.

B_5, or pantothenic acid, participates in the release of energy from the digestion of carbohydrates, fats, and proteins, and it aids in the utilization of vitamins. It helps build cells; aids in the maintenance of the nervous system and the immune system; maintains healthy skin; supports the adrenal glands, which produce cortisol in times of stress; fights infection by building antibodies; detoxifies the body; stimulates growth; and helps the body to utilize vitamin D.

B_5 deficiencies can result in asthma attacks, muscle cramping, painful and burning feet, skin abnormalities, retarded growth, dizzy spells, weakness, depression, decreased resistance to infection, restlessness, digestive disturbances, and vomiting.

Vitamin B_6, also known as pyridoxine or pyridoxal phosphate, is necessary for the synthesis and breakdown of amino acids. It is required by the central nervous system for the normal functioning of the brain. B_6 also aids in the metabolism of fat and carbohydrates, the formation of antibodies, and the removal of excess fluid and lessening of discomfort during the menstrual period. It aids hemoglobin in its function; promotes healthy skin; reduces muscle spasms, leg cramps, and stiffness of the hands; helps to prevent nausea; and promotes the balance of sodium and phosphorus in the body.

Conditions that respond to B_6 therapy include carpal tunnel syndrome, joint pain, homocystinuria, sensitivity to bright light, sensitivity to MSG, burning or tingling in the extremities, the inability to recall dreams, and imbalances of the liver. Because vitamin B_6 is used by the body to break down protein, the more protein one eats, the more vitamin B_6 one needs. Deficiencies can produce skin eruptions, loss of muscular control or muscle weakness, arm and leg cramps, fatigue, nervousness, irritability, insomnia, slow learning, water retention, anemia, mouth disorders, or hair loss.

Good sources of B_6 are meat, poultry, fish, fruits, vegetables, and grain products. Most ready-to-eat and instant cereals are fortified with B_6. To retain B_6 during cooking, serve fruits raw, cook vegetables in a minimal amount of water for the shortest time possible, and roast or broil meat and poultry.

Vitamin B_{12}, also known as cobalamin or cyanocobalamin, is required for the formation and regeneration of red blood cells to help prevent anemia. B_{12} is also necessary for building genetic material, producing energy, maintaining a healthy nervous system and muscles, and metabolizing carbohydrates, fat, and protein. It is important for the promotion of DNA synthesis, childhood growth, cell longevity, memory improvement, maintenance of the appetite and digestive system, and strengthening of the immune system. It aids in the absorption of iron and calcium and helps prevent inflammation. It also assists in folate metabolism and in the synthesis of DNA, and is essential to producing insulation for nerve fibers. B_{12}

and a coenzyme form dibencozide, which aids in the conversion of fat to lean muscle tissue. For this reason many athletes, such as weight lifters, take B_{12} as a safe, competitive, and legal alternative to steroids. A B_{12}-folate complex can be used as a tonic to assist in the conversion of iron to hemoglobin, to help normalize hormonal production, and to improve short-term memory in the elderly. B_{12} is even considered an antiaging nutrient and an agent for increasing sperm count. B_{12} should not be taken indiscriminately in high doses, so check with your physician and/or nutritionist on how much B_{12} you may need to take each day.

There is some controversy today about the best way to get enough B_{12} in our diets. The standard belief is that B_{12} is found naturally only in animal foods—meat, eggs, and milk products. But a number of vegetarians and vegans claim they have found numerous nonanimal sources of this vital nutrient, including edible seaweeds such as hijiki and wakame, certain mushrooms, sourdough bread, tofu, tempeh, miso, barley malt syrup, parsley, beer, cider, wine, and margarine. Some nutritionists disagree, however, saying that the only food sources of B_{12} available to vegetarians are fortified nutritional yeast, fortified breakfast cereals, soy milk, and other soy products.

Supplements that contain spirulina or nori can interfere with B_{12} absorption. Some experts also advise against taking multivitamin products because these may contain substances that interfere with the breakdown of B_{12}. By preventing the absorption of B_{12}, they help to create the deficiency they are supposed to correct.

B_{12} can be produced by bacterial activity in the body's own small intestine, mouth, and nasal passages, and around the tonsils and upper bronchial tree. Since B_{12} is often found in soil, freshly picked vegetables, especially root vegetables, may have B_{12} on their surfaces. To retain the B_{12} in meat or fish, these foods should be roasted or broiled.

A person deficient in B_{12} could experience pernicious anemia, degeneration of the spinal cord and nerves, poor appetite, stunted growth, nervousness, depression, lack of balance, neuritis, or brain damage. Symptoms of anemia might include an abnormally pale, yellow, or sallow complexion; a shiny or sore and red tongue; weakness and fatigue that progresses to paralysis; numbness or tingling in the hands and feet; gradual deterioration of motor coordination; moodiness; poor memory and confusion; and even delirium, delusion, hallucinations, and psychotic states. Paralysis and possible death may occur with the deterioration of the myelin sheaths that surround nerves and the failure of DNA production.

A B_{12} deficiency, especially among the elderly, may occur even though the person's diet contains enough of this vitamin. This is because other substances needed for B_{12} absorption might be lacking. For example, the stomach manufactures something known as intrinsic factor, which must bond with B_{12} before the body can absorb it. Other substances that are needed for the absorption of this vitamin include iron and folic acid. Microorganisms in the stomach can compete for the available supply of B_{12}, and toxins can block absorption. Enzyme deficiencies, liver or kidney disease, and atrophic gastritis can interfere with the utilization of B_{12}.

B_{12} can be further depleted by hypothyroidism and an allergy to lactose. Consumption of meat and animal products (including eggs), refined sugars, carbohydrates, drugs, caffeine, alcoholic beverages, tobacco, and megadoses of vitamin C—and allergies to any of these foods—can all use up the body's store of B_{12}.

Sufficient levels of B_{12} are considered especially crucial for women during pregnancy and lactation. The best source of B_{12} is organ meat, such as heart, liver, and kidney. Clams, oysters, beef, port wine, eggs, and milk are also good sources of B_{12}.

Folic acid (folate or folicin) helps the body form red blood cells and aids in the formation of genetic material within every body cell. Folic acid also works with vitamin B_{12} in synthesizing DNA and RNA, which is essential for the growth and reproduction of all body cells. It is useful in amino acid conversion (the breakdown and assimilation of protein), stimulation of the appetite, maintenance of a healthy intestinal tract, and the formation of nucleic acid. Folic acid may reverse certain types of anemia, reduce the risk of cervical dysplasia, and lower the likelihood of a heart attack. It becomes even more essential during times of growth and cell reproduction, especially during pregnancy, when it can protect the fetus against neural tube defects such as spina bifida, which can cause permanent crippling. Recently it was discovered that folic acid reduces the risk of premature birth.

A deficiency in folic acid can also result in megaloblastic anemia, a disease in which red blood cells fail to divide properly, becoming large and abnormal. Other symptoms of folic acid deficiency are gastrointestinal disorders, prematurely gray hair, a pale tongue, and vitamin B_{12} deficiency.

To retain folic acid, fruits and vegetables should be eaten raw, if possible, or steamed or simmered in a minimal amount of water. Always store your vegetables in the refrigerator. Good sources of folic acid include citrus fruits, tomatoes, green leafy vegetables, broccoli, grain products, and organ meats.

Biotin is another B vitamin that the body needs for optimal health. Biotin helps to strengthen the immune system. It also aids in the utilization of protein, folic acid, pantothenic acid, and vitamin B_{12}; aids in cell growth and fatty acid production; helps in the formation of DNA and RNA; and helps to produce healthy hair.

Anyone who is allergic to this particular B vitamin will not be able to properly absorb it or any of the other B vitamins. A biotin deficiency may lead to drowsiness, extreme exhaustion, depression, loss of appetite, muscle pain, and grayish skin.

Inositol, found in every cell of the body, is necessary for the growth of muscle cells and the formation of lecithin. It aids in the breakdown of fats, helps reduce blood cholesterol, and helps prevent hair loss. Inositol is also a free-radical scavenger and is known as "nature's tranquilizer" for the calming effect it often has. A deficiency may result in hair loss, eczema, constipation, migraines, and high cholesterol.

Choline is very important in controlling fat and cholesterol buildup in the body, preventing fat from accumulating in the liver, and facilitating the movement of fats in the cells and throughout the bloodstream. It also helps regulate the function of the kidneys, liver, and gallbladder. It is important in maintaining the health of the myelin sheaths covering the nerves, and in facilitating nerve transmission. Choline is known to help improve memory and support brain chemistry, and it is an essential component of acetylcholine, an important neurotransmitter.

A deficiency in this vitamin may result in cirrhosis and fatty degeneration of the liver, hardening of the arteries, heart problems, high blood pressure, and hemorrhaging kidneys. Choline should be taken with the other B vitamins for optimal effectiveness.

Para-aminobenzoic acid (PABA) is a component of folic acid as well as an antioxidant and membrane stabilizer. It helps to prevent red blood cells from bursting and lysosomal membranes from breaking and releasing tissue-damaging enzymes. PABA helps bacteria to produce folic acid and aids in the formation of red blood cells and the assimilation of pantothenic acid. When used externally it produces healthy skin and skin pigmentation, helps return gray hair to its natural color, and screens the skin from sun exposure. A PABA deficiency may cause extreme fatigue, irritability, depression, nervousness, eczema, constipation, digestive disorders, headaches, and premature graying of hair.

ALLERGIES TO VITAMIN A

Another essential vitamin that people experience allergies to is vitamin A. When people are allergic to vitamin A, they may not be able to absorb it. Vitamin A and beta-carotene, which is converted to vitamin A in the body, are important immune system stimulants and protective agents that are crucial for healthy mucous membranes, and the prevention of respiratory infections and skin eruptions. Many physicians recommend vitamin A supplements for asthma sufferers as well as for those with skin disorders, which is fine as long as you are not allergic to it. A vitamin A deficiency can disturb white blood cell production in the body and lower immune function. It is necessary for maintaining good vision and preventing night blindness, skin disorders, colds, influenza, and other infections. It helps heal ulcers and wounds and is necessary for the growth of bones and teeth. Vitamin A is an antioxidant and helps protect the cells against free radicals. Beta-carotene, which is found in vegetables, is good for the prevention of chronic health problems and is a powerful anti-oxidant.

A deficiency in vitamin A can cause skin tags, warts, blemishes, acne, rashes, hair loss, and premature aging. Inadequate intake can also cause increased bronchial, lung, and respiratory problems, lowered immunity, infertility, joint pain, vomiting, and gastrointestinal problems. Vitamin A works in conjunction with other nutrients; B vitamins, vitamins D and E, calcium, and zinc are needed to mobilize it from the liver, where it is stored. Large doses of vitamin A should be taken only under proper supervision because it can accumulate to toxic levels in the body. Similarly, people who are allergic to vitamin A and ingest large amounts that they are unable to absorb risk accumulating toxic levels in the liver. After this allergy is cleared, however, supplementation may be helpful for a period of time.

A vitamin A allergy may be implicated in allergies to such foods as papayas, peaches, asparagus, beets, broccoli, carrots, Swiss chard, kale, turnip greens, watercress, parsley, red peppers, sweet potatoes, squash, pumpkin, corn, spirulina, milk, butter, other dairy products, egg yolk, fish, and fish liver oil.

∾ JOSHUA'S STORY

At my clinic, I recently worked with a four-year-old boy named Joshua who suffered from chronic ear infections. He had been on and off antibiotics for over a year. Under another physician's recommendations, he supplemented with high doses of vitamins A and C, but continued to get ear infections. After thorough investigation and testing, I noticed that Joshua consistently experienced nausea soon after ingesting his vitamin A supplement. For this reason, I suspected that vitamin A might be a major allergen for him. I recommended to Joshua's mother that the vitamin A supplements be discontinued until an allergy elimination treatment could be performed, and she agreed. After the first level of allergy treatments was done, I treated Joshua for vitamin A. His strong reaction to this vitamin cleared and he was able to begin supplementing it in a formulation that included enzymes. Joshua has been symptom free for nine months and continues to do well.

I also experienced a major allergic reaction to vitamin A, both as a young child and into adulthood. For this reason, I was unable to eat carrots, a food high in vitamin A, since they would immediately trigger a severe headache, even when I ate small amounts. During my initial development of BioSET™, I was tested for a vitamin A allergy and, sure enough, I had one. Soon afterward I was treated for vitamin A with the BioSET™ allergy elimination technique, and now I can eat carrots every day with no adverse reactions.

VITAMIN E

Vitamin E is a fat-soluble antioxidant vitamin that protects cells from free-radical damage and neutralizes the damaging effects of ozone. An allergy to vitamin E can result in allergies to foods such as wheat germ or wheat germ oil, vegetable oils, soybeans or soybean oil, green vegetables, flours, grains, eggs, raw nuts or sprouted seeds, and fish.

ESSENTIAL FATTY ACIDS

Fats, or fatty acids, are needed for the absorption of vitamins A, D, K, and beta-carotene. An allergy to fatty acids can reduce the integrity of cell membranes, weaken the nervous system, and impact the immune system's ability to help ward off disease. Fat also helps slow the release of sugar into the bloodstream, so a fat allergy contributes to hypoglycemia and can affect diabetics.

Allergies to animal fats and vegetable oils have been known to promote estrogen secretion in the body, causing increased menopausal and premenstrual symptoms, as well as premenstrual headaches and menstrual cramping. Allergies to these foods can also cause excess weight gain, increased arthritic pain, and constipation.

Of all the fats we consume, there are only a few essential fatty acids. They fall into two classes: omega-6 fatty acids and omega-3 fatty acids. Omega-6 fatty acids can be found in all vegetable oils and in most grains and beans. Omega-3s are found in fewer foods: flaxseed, flaxseed oil, fresh walnuts, walnut oil, pumpkin seeds, and soy and canola oils.

Both of these fats can be used to fight inflammation, as researchers have repeatedly shown. Inflammation is controlled by various chemicals in your body, but the most important are prostaglandins. Prostaglandins are potent stimulators of muscle contraction and vasodilation. Your body manufactures these prostaglandins from the fats you eat, especially the fats found in meats and cooking oils. Prostaglandin E2 causes tissues to swell following an injury. Two different prostaglandins, E1 and E3, have the opposite effect—they reduce inflammation by blocking swelling, pain, redness, and heat. Fats high in omega-3 fatty acids turn into prostaglandin E1 and E3, reduce inflammation, and therefore can benefit those with arthritic symptoms. People with arthritis may have allergies to these fatty acids.

It is important to keep oils fresh, as rancidity destroys the healthy essential fatty acids. Avoid buying oils sold in clear bottles, as the oil becomes rancid more quickly. Tinted glass bottles, such as the ones that olive oils are often sold in, and the dark plastic containers in which flaxseed oil is sold help prevent rancidity. Also, do not store oils in the pantry for long periods of time.

IRON

Iron is an essential nutrient that aids in growth, promotes resistance to disease, and prevents fatigue. Like calcium, however, it can be a potential allergen. People with an iron allergy may become anemic or suffer from other chronic iron deficiency problems. Allergic reactions may include backaches, headaches, dizziness, menstrual problems, and fatigue. Physicians may try to treat deficiencies by prescribing iron supplements for long periods of time, but quite often the results are not favorable because the allergy prevents proper absorption of this mineral.

Clearing this allergy may clear allergies to many foods that contain iron, including apricots, peaches, bananas, prunes, raisins, blackstrap molasses, brewer's yeast, whole grains, cereals, turnip greens, spinach, beets, beet greens, alfalfa, asparagus, kelp, sunflower seeds, walnuts, sesame seeds, beans, egg yolk, liver, red meat, oysters, and clams.

MAGNESIUM

Magnesium is another mineral to which people might be allergic. There has been considerable study regarding the use of magnesium as a treatment for asthmatics and migraine sufferers, but I have commonly found it necessary to treat clients for a magnesium allergy before supplementing. Once the allergy is cleared, magnesium can be helpful in reducing asthma episodes and greatly inhibiting migraines. Magnesium is found in nuts and seeds, soybeans, green leafy vegetables, and whole grains.

Magnesium is a smooth-muscle relaxant and can work magically to eliminate severe asthma attacks. It is also a natural laxative and therefore extremely helpful with chronic constipation.

A study in Britain tested over 2,500 adults using a chemical that is known to constrict the airways in asthmatic sufferers. They found that people with diets low in magnesium were twice as likely to have an adverse reaction to this substance than those with high-magnesium diets. Another study, in France, found that asthmatics have lower levels of magnesium in the tissues of their airways than do people without asthma. This study spurred further research into the anti-inflammatory properties of magnesium.

ZINC

The mineral zinc is a key nutrient in skin health, and a zinc allergy can be responsible for eczema and acne. Zinc is found in green leafy vegetables, pork, beef, lamb, fish, brown rice, eggs, milk, brewer's yeast, mushrooms, onions, peas, dried beans, seeds, wheat bran, wheat germ, herring, oysters, and mustard.

SUGARS

Sugar allergies affect all of us. In fact, I rarely find a person who is not allergic to sugars. Sugars are implicated in many different health problems, such as chronic deficiencies in the immune system, accumulation of mucus in the throat and respiratory system, malabsorption of vitamins and minerals, indigestion, mood swings, weight problems, arthritis, muscle and joint pain, and depression. Sugars come in many types; check food labels for terms such as *maltose, glucose, dextrose, lactose, fructose, brown sugar, honey, corn sugar, raw sugar, cane sugar, molasses, high-fructose corn syrup, grape sugar,* and *maple sugar.* A list of foods containing sugars is in Appendix 2.

Sugar allergies can cause cravings for foods high in sugar, such as cookies, cakes, pastries, and ice cream. Clearing a sugar allergy with the BioSET™ allergy elimination technique can reduce those cravings. Reducing food cravings can profoundly benefit a weight loss routine, prevent tooth decay, improve behavioral and attention problems in children, and reduce mood swings. Clearing a sugar allergy can eliminate a child's battle with chronic ear infections, sore throats, or sinus congestion. Asthmatics with chronic coughs stop coughing, sometimes overnight, with this technique. Joint pain can be obliterated within ten days after a sugar clearing.

✑✐ CLAIRE'S STORY

Claire, a sixty-seven-year-old woman, came to my office with severe hip and knee pain. She was also sixty pounds overweight. She wanted very much to lose weight but had not been successful with any of the weight loss regimes she had tried over the past few years, and she wondered if food allergies could be a factor. She also confessed that she had voracious sugar cravings, a common reaction to foods to which one is allergic.

Her allergy testing revealed many food allergies, and sugar allergies were among the most severe. I recommended a sugar/starch digestive enzyme, as well as my sugar-intolerant diet, which you will find in Chapter 11. I also began treating her with BioSET™ allergy treatments.

After the first treatment, Claire noticed some improvement in her joint pain and reported that some of her food cravings were slightly improved. She was hopeful and ready to clear the sugar allergy. On her second visit Claire was treated for sugars. Two weeks later she skipped into my office, literally. She was pain free, her joints were more flexible, and she had lost thirteen pounds. She had committed herself to my sugar-intolerant diet, which had completely eliminated her sugar cravings, and she had started walking three miles every morning. She was ecstatic. At the end of three months of care, Claire had returned to her normal weight and was feeling very happy. Her daughter also became a patient for weight loss and is currently doing very well.

SODIUM

Clearing an allergy to sodium can also be a significant step in clearing allergies to other foods. Foods high in sodium include watermelon, celery, pineapples, kelp, shellfish, and processed foods. Sodium allergies can cause water retention, high blood pressure, headaches, and coughs. A recent study suggests a correlation between levels of sodium intake and asthma symptoms, especially among men. High sodium intake is also correlated with deaths from asthma in men and children. Other studies have shown an increased bronchial activity in men with high sodium intake, but not in women.

PHENOLICS AND BIOCHEMICALS

The next priority in identifying food allergies is to understand and learn to identify phenolics and biochemicals in foods. (I define biochemicals as chemicals found in foods.) Phenolics, found in many foods, are a class of aromatic compounds that have in common a specific chemical called benzene. Phenolics give foods much of their flavor and aroma, and can also be added to foods to help prevent spoilage. Some phenolics help in the germination of seeds, and others protect plants against invaders such as insects and molds.

Phenolics and biochemicals should always be cleared before you attempt to clear any food by itself. The reason for this is that most food allergies are usually eliminated through these clearings. If these clearings aren't completely successful in desensitizing your food allergies, clearing specific vitamins, minerals, and sugar will most often complete the picture.

There are several phenolics and biochemicals commonly found in foods, including caffeine, vanillin, cinnamic acid, and limonene, but there are others that are less frequently encountered. When I treat someone for food allergies, I usually treat for phenolics and biochemicals together; later in this book I will explain how you can do this at home.

✐ DORIS'S STORY

Doris, a woman in her late fifties, suffered severe reactions to many foods, including almost all grains except rice, all dairy products, all meats and fish, and all vegetables. Doris subsisted on only chicken, some beans, and fruit. But sometimes, due to circumstances beyond her control, she would find herself eating the things to which she was allergic. Within two hours of eating these provoking foods, she would generally experience fatigue, dizziness, a headache, flatulence, and nausea. She came to me with the hope that someday she could eat normally and not experience these symptoms.

Doris's food allergies had begun about ten years previously, and she had tried many different therapies, all of which had proven ineffective. Her friend Mindy, a patient of another BioSET™ practitioner, had had enormous success being cured from her chronic hay fever and sinus congestion, and referred Doris to my office.

Doris's first visit consisted of an enzyme evaluation examination and allergy testing. The enzyme evaluation revealed a severe protein intolerance, making it impossible for her to digest most proteins. I recommended that she take an enzyme to support her digestion. I also recommended the protein-intolerant diet, found in Chapter 11. That same afternoon I tested her for allergies and noted that she was allergic to most foods and many phenolics. I told Doris that, based on my years of experience, I was certain that her food allergies would clear after she was desensitized to the phenolics and amino acids. Doris was glad to hear this and eager to begin our work. First I cleared the phenolics; two weeks later, when I retested her, I found no sensitivity, and subsequently a complete food allergy retest showed that she was allergy free. She told me that she was able to eat all of her favorite foods again, including wheat bread, Parmesan cheese, broccoli, carrots, and steak, with absolutely no symptoms.

Doris is one of thousands of patients for whom this has been the outcome. This is exactly what I want readers to appreciate and learn to accomplish for themselves. You can all experience freedom from food allergies.

AMINO ACIDS

Clearing for amino acids can also be useful in curing many food allergies, since most foods, except lettuce, have one or many amino acids in them. Some of the amino acids I have found significant as causes of food allergies are listed in the following chart.

AMINO ACID	FOUND IN	SYMPTOMS OF ALLERGY
Alanine	Wheat germ, ricotta and cottage cheese, turkey, duck	Candida, connective tissue disorders, diabetes
Arginine	Algae, spirulina, meat, nuts, eggs, cheese, seeds, peas, chocolate, garlic, ginseng	Premature aging, autism, collagen diseases, fatigue, headaches, high cholesterol level, learning disabilities, retarded growth, underweight, urinary incontinence
Asparagine	Pollen, seeds, plants	Headaches
Carnitine	Red meat, lamb, pork, avocadoes, human breast milk	Angina, heart problems, decreased energy, being overweight, muscle weakness
Citrulline	Watermelon, onions, scallions, garlic	Fatigue, migraine
Glutamic acid	Oatmeal, wheat gluten, granola, cheese, cottage cheese, whole milk, chocolate, eggs, avocadoes, peaches, ham, bacon, chicken, duck, turkey, wild game	Premature aging, autism, bloating and flatulence, diarrhea, celiac disease, colitis, depression, dyskinesia, fatigue, hypertension, hypoglycemia, migraine headache, nausea, nervousness, sinusitis, sugar cravings

(continued)

AMINO ACID	FOUND IN	SYMPTOMS OF ALLERGY
Glutamine	Celery root, sugar beets, carrots, radishes	Autism, bloating, diarrhea, fatigue, food cravings, hyperactivity, hypoglycemia, learning difficulties, memory and concentration problems, migraines, nervousness, sinusitis
Glycine	Sugarcane, wheat germ, pork, chicken, turkey, duck, wild game, sausage, avocadoes	Connective tissue weakness, fatigue, fibrocystic disease, hyperactivity, inability to heal, retarded growth, seizures, mental problems
Hydroxylysine	Gelatin	Premature aging of skin, pain in limbs
Leucine	Wheat germ, cottage cheese and ricotta, pork, sausage, chicken, turkey, duck, soy protein, fish, eggs, legumes, whole wheat, beans, nuts, seeds	Anxiety, depression, edema, retarded growth, susceptibility to infection, irritability, menstrual problems, nightmares, pain
Lysine	Grains, seeds, nuts, dairy products, meats, yeast	Learning disabilities, recurring herpes, stomach pain, susceptibility to viral infections
Methionine	Sunflower seeds, wheat germ, ricotta, pork, chicken, duck, turkey, avocadoes, cheeses	Eczema, gum problems, bloating, constipation, bad breath, food cravings, psoriasis, schizophrenia
Phenylalanine	Eggs, milk, wild rice, beef, chicken, fish, eggs, soybeans, cottage cheese, baked beans, bananas, peanuts, almonds	Arthritis, blurred vision, headache, chest problems, depression, gas, hyperactivity, hypertension, itching of mouth, learning disabilities, lupus, Parkinson's disease, respiratory congestion, severe weakness, shoulder pain,

AMINO ACID	FOUND IN	SYMPTOMS OF ALLERGY
		sleep problems, sugar cravings
Proline	Gliadin, gelatin	Fatigue, weak fingernails, headaches, premature aging
Taurine	Animal protein, mussels, oysters	Atherosclerosis, candida, chemical sensitivities, epilepsy, headaches, hypertension, insomnia, mental problems, seizures, Tourette's syndrome
Threonine	Eggs, skim milk, casein, gelatin, oats, wheat germ, ricotta, cottage cheese, pork, chicken, turkey, duck, wild game	Fatigue
Tyrosine	Milk, casein, corn, pork, turkey, duck	Adrenal insufficiency, headaches, hypothyroid symptoms, obesity, parkinsonism-type symptoms, restless legs, sleep disorders
Valine	Soy, raw brown rice, cottage cheese, fish, beef, lamb, chicken, nuts, lentils, mushrooms	Premature aging, fatigue, hallucinations, migraines, sleepiness, lack of muscle stamina

Like the clearing of phenolics, clearing allergies to amino acids is an essential step in clearing food allergies. And as you can see in the chart above, there are many symptoms related to amino acid allergies. I have found that a patient's negative reaction to a certain food might actually signal an allergy to an essential amino acid that is superabundant in the foods one eats regularly. That is why I was not surprised when Joseph, a twenty-five-year-old student, was relieved of severe nightmares after I cleared him for amino acids. I have many other patients who were cured of a variety of symptoms after being desensitized to amino acids. Jill, a five-year-old girl, ceased having seizures. Rob, age fifty-three, was freed from his severe sugar cravings and his two-year battle with hypertension. A nineteen-year-old woman named Susan won her battle against bulimia and anorexia. Lana was able to finally become pregnant. Clearing amino acids is a requisite to successfully eliminate food allergies.

ENZYMES

A deficiency of enzymes can also be a root cause of food intolerances. If you lack one or more enzymes, you may experience digestive problems such as diarrhea and stomach pain after consuming foods that the missing enzyme digests. For example, people who have difficulty drinking milk frequently are allergic to the enzyme that digests lactose, a sugar found in milk. In my clinical practice I have found that people who are lactose intolerant can essentially be cleared of that reaction by undergoing the BioSET™ allergy elimination treatment.

COMMON FOODS THAT CAN TRIGGER ALLERGIES

DAIRY PRODUCTS

An allergy to dairy products such as milk, yogurt, and cheese is one of the most common and widely recognized food allergies. I have found that dairy allergies can often be eliminated by clearing calcium, lactose, amino acids, and phenolics. Occasionally, however, it is important to treat for the actual dairy product itself. With a combination of BioSET™ treatment and enzyme therapy, dairy intolerance can be eliminated.

One of the most usual complaints associated with a dairy product allergy is excess mucus production. Probably all of us have had this kind of experience at some time or another—the need to clear our throats after eating a certain food. I remember one woman who constantly had mucus in her throat, especially after she ate dairy products. After we treated her with BioSET™, she no longer had this problem with any food, including dairy. She was surprised at this because, like many of us, she believed that dairy products are always mucus-producing. Before working with this method of clearing, I had believed the same thing, and I was equally surprised by our results. Other symptoms associated with dairy products are arthritis pain and swelling, and digestive problems ranging from bloating to severe diarrhea.

EGGS

Many people are highly allergic to eggs and chicken. I have found that 90 percent of the time, clearing amino acids will eliminate an egg allergy. But these foods might also require specific treatment. When my daughter, Gabrielle, was two years old, she began experiencing chronic mucus in her throat, making it necessary for her to clear her throat on a regular basis. This symptom became more apparent as she grew older, and by age three she began to comment about it.

At the same time, she also craved eggs and would often go into the refrigerator, take out an egg, and ask me to prepare it for her. As you remember, food cravings usually point toward an allergy to that food. When I treated her for amino acids using BioSET™, her egg craving disappeared, and so did her chronic mucus condition.

Eggs can also be implicated in arthritis and headaches.

SOY PRODUCTS

Soybeans are an excellent source of protein. Soy products also contain weak plant estrogens called phytoestrogens that bind to estrogen-sensitive cells, thus reducing the number of sites natural estrogen can attach to. By binding to estrogen receptors, phytoestrogens may limit the effects of environmental estrogens and estrogen-like substances. And plant estrogens might also help to reduce menopausal symptoms. For this reason, many women begin adding soy to their diet as they enter their premenopausal years. So taking soy may also reduce or eliminate the need for estrogen replacement drug therapy, commonly recommended to postmenopausal women; estrogen replacement can cause gallbladder disease and abnormal blood clotting. Clots can cause a stroke, heart attack, or pulmonary embolism, any of which can be fatal. Estrogen is likely to produce uncomfortable side effects such as nausea and vomiting. It can enlarge breasts and make them tender. Women who take estrogen can also retain excess fluid, which can aggravate conditions such as asthma, epilepsy, migraines, and heart and kidney disease. A spotty darkening of the skin, particularly on the face, can be caused by this hormone.

But instead of reaping the benefits of soy, women are often bogged down by allergic reactions to this food. In fact, most women I test are allergic to soy and need to be treated for it. Many mothers who bring their children to me because of chronic ear infections or eczema inform me that they removed cow's milk from the children's diet and began substituting soy milk. Although these mothers mean well, this practice may result in children who develop chronic upper respiratory infections or increased eczema because they are allergic to soy. Other symptoms commonly caused by soy include severe bloating, gas, and asthma.

Soy is a main ingredient in many nondairy milk and cheese products, nonwheat flours, and many types of vegetarian "meats," with new products coming out all the time. Soy lecithin is often used in candy to prevent drying and to help emulsify the fats, so clearing lecithin can often help clear a chocolate sensitivity. Soy is also used in many other foods where you might not expect it. Soy flour is used in hard candies, fudge, nut candies, and caramels. Some bakeries use soy milk instead of cow's milk in recipes, and soy products are used in custards.

Soy products may also be used in household products such as varnish, paints, enamels, printing ink, massage creams, celluloid, paper finishes, cloth, nitroglycerin, pet food, adhesives, soap, fertilizer, automobile parts, textiles, and lubricating oil. Ford Motor Company has used soybeans to make a plastic for window frames, steering wheels, and other automotive parts. It even uses soy to make a rubber substitute and an upholstery fabric. As soy becomes more common in the environment, it is important that sensitive people be treated for it.

GRAINS

Corn is a major grain allergen. In fact, it may be one of the most common allergies today. Many foods and products you might not suspect contain corn. Cornstarch is found in Chinese food, baking powder, and toothpaste, and it is the binding product in most tablets, including aspirin, Tylenol, and other kinds of drugs. Corn syrup is a common sweetener found in many soft drinks. You can find corn oil in food mixes, canned foods, and fried foods. And corn silk is used in several makeup products. Corn allergies can cause migraines, arthritis, and digestive problems.

A wheat allergy, especially if coupled with a corn allergy, can cause severe health problems. Wheat allergies can cause symptoms ranging from fatigue to eczema, arthritis, digestive problems, colitis, food cravings, and brain fog. I have been very successful in completely clearing wheat allergies by treating for allergies to maltose (a sugar that occurs naturally in wheat), B vitamins, amino acids, and phenolics. Foods that contain wheat are so numerous that I have listed them in Appendix 2.

Barley, oats, and rye can also be allergens. I have had success clearing these grains by initially treating for phenolics and then gluten. Allergies to these grains result in symptoms of the digestive system (bloating and gas) and skin (dry skin and eczema).

FRUITS

Any fruit can be a potential allergen. I have seen people who are allergic to just about all of them, including apples, bananas, grapes, pears, melons, pineapples, strawberries, kiwis, papayas, and mangoes. Many children drink an enormous amount of apple juice, which can be mucus-forming if they are allergic to it. Bananas can have the same effect. Consequently, both apple juice and bananas can be a particular problem for asthmatics. The chemicals that are sprayed on fruit can also be a problem for people and can trigger serious responses in asthmatics.

Treating for vitamin C, bioflavonoids, sugars, and phenolics can often clear fruit allergies.

PEANUTS

Peanuts, a common allergen, are widely used in many food products. The incidence of peanut allergy has risen in the last decade, perhaps because of the increased use of peanut products and peanut butter as a source of protein. Research has indicated that many mothers use peanut butter to supplement their protein intake while breast-feeding. Because peanut allergens are secreted in breast milk, this can create a sensitivity to this substance in an at-risk child.

Reactions from peanuts include mucus formation, asthmatic attacks, and anaphylactic shock. An anaphylactic allergy is beyond the scope of this book and any home clearing, so seek out a professional if you experience that response. A peanut allergy can also induce migraines and digestive problems, which can be cleared with the BioSET™ method. Clearing for phenolics can often successfully clear this allergen. Other nuts to watch out for are cashews, pecans, and walnuts.

PLANTS IN THE NIGHTSHADE FAMILY

Eggplants, potatoes, tomatoes, and peppers are all members of the nightshade family. Any of them can be serious allergens and can provoke immediate allergic reactions. Nightshades can act as irritants for those with arthritis or joint pain and can induce migraines and cause digestive problems. Sometimes a condition that has been diagnosed as arthritis is actually an allergy to one of these foods. Studies have indicated that an allergy to eggplant is linked to allergies to grasses, ragweed, birch, and animal dander.

VEGETABLES

Other vegetables besides those in the nightshade family are potential allergens. Onions have always been known as a common trigger for asthmatics. Yams, cucumbers, and carrots are sometimes a problem. These are the most common vegetable allergies I have encountered. Carrots can be a powerful allergen, inducing asthma, migraines, or severe skin eczema.

Treating for vitamin A will often clear a sensitivity to carrots without having to clear the carrots themselves.

Allergies to dried beans can cause digestive problems, headaches, or migraines. The beans people are most often allergic to are garbanzo, kidney, and pinto beans. Clearing phenolics will usually clear this allergy very easily.

SEAFOOD

Fish and shellfish can cause severe allergic reactions, including eczema, asthma, migraines, digestive problems, sinus congestion, gout, and arthritis.

CHOCOLATE, CAFFEINE, AND COFFEE

Chocolate and caffeine are common allergens. A craving for chocolate is usually indicative of a chocolate allergy. Caffeine is found in obvious sources such as coffee and tea and is also a hidden ingredient in some soft drinks and over-the-counter medications such as Excedrin. An allergy to caffeine or chocolate can cause migraines, arthritis pain, heartburn and reflux, breast tenderness, an increased tendency to develop endometriosis, asthma, coughing, and sinus congestion. Coffee, tea, and caffeine can usually be cleared through a phenolics treatment. When a forty-two-year-old woman named Jean came to my office complaining of a chronic cough, her coughing stopped immediately after I had treated her for caffeine as part of the phenolics protocol.

SPICES

Allergies to certain types of spices are very common. Garlic is a common allergen, although it is regarded by many as a healthy food. I have seen asthmatics who begin wheezing after eating excessive amounts of garlic. It can also cause indigestion, bloating, and headaches. Other spices I commonly find to be allergens are cinnamon, cardamom, curry, dill, ginger, mustard, oregano, paprika, black pepper, cayenne pepper, rosemary, sage, and tarragon.

SALICYLATES

Salicylates are chemicals that are both found naturally in foods and added as a preservative. Salicylates can cause asthma, digestive problems, nasal congestion, sleep problems, tongue lesions, and hyperactivity. Most sensitive individuals will not react to salicylates every time they are eaten unless they are consumed in excessive amounts, so usually foods containing these chemicals can be tolerated in a rotation diet, but not if eaten daily.

Salicylates are found in a variety of fruits, including apples, apricots, blackberries, boysenberries, cantaloupe, cherries, cranberries, currants, dates, guavas, grapes, loganberries, oranges, pineapples, plums, raspberries, strawberries, and gooseberries. They are also found in chicory, hot and sweet peppers, endives, mushrooms, radishes, tomato sauce, zucchini, almonds, peanuts, water chestnuts, bay leaves, basil, caraway, ginger, mint, nutmeg, cloves, green olives, champagne, white pepper, peppermint, port wine, tea (black and herbal), vanilla extract, and wine vinegar. A variety of crackers, some cereals, cake mixes, muffins, biscuits, cakes, coffee, pastries, tobacco, mayonnaise, ketchup, Jell-O and gelatin, candies, gum, and corned beef have salicylates added to them as well. Aspirin also contains salicylates.

FOOD ADDITIVES

Many food additives can cause allergic reactions. These include sulfites, MSG, hydrolyzed vegetable protein, and sodium nitrite. Sulfites in particular are potentially deadly for asthmatics. I have seen several cases of children who had a serious reaction after eating fast foods containing sulfites. Sulfites are used as preservatives in salad bars and shellfish bars. They are also found in wines, both red and white.

Most food additives are listed on the labels of prepared foods, but small amounts of substances do not, by law, have to be mentioned. For this reason, sensitive people can eat something they are allergic to without being aware of it. Preservatives such as BHA and BHT, which are used in packaging, may cause reactions in sensitive people who eat the food contained in that packaging.

MSG has been used for many years as a flavor enhancer for a variety of foods prepared at home and in restaurants. MSG is manufactured by a fermentation process that uses starch, beet sugar, cane sugar, or molasses and a sodium salt of glutamic acid (an amino acid that is found naturally in our bodies and also constitutes a large part of the proteins found in foods such as cheese, meat, peas, mushrooms, and milk). MSG can cause migraines, visual disturbances, erratic behavior, asthma, hives, and severe anaphylactic reactions.

The FDA has studied many of the reportedly adverse effects of MSG, but unfortunately still considers it a safe ingredient. I disagree. I treat many people who are allergic to MSG and find that it causes particular problems for asthmatics.

Any packaged food containing MSG as a separate ingredient must say so on the label. You can look for MSG in dips, soup mixes, stews, gravy, sauces, and prepared meats, poultry, fish, and vegetables. In restaurants that claim they do not use MSG or will not add it to your food upon request, you might still get MSG in the commercial sauces or spice mixes that they use.

People who are allergic to MSG may be allergic to other glutamate products as well. Be aware that MSG and the other glutamates do *not* have to be listed separately as ingredients if they are a component of another commonly used ingredient, such as hydrolyzed vegetable protein. This can have serious consequences for people who are allergic and have no way of knowing that they are eating these additives. Food ingredients that contain glutamate include hydrolyzed vegetable protein, autolyzed yeast, some extract flavorings and other natural flavorings, and potassium glutamate. Hydrolyzed vegetable protein contains 5 to 20 percent glutamate and is used in place of MSG as a flavor enhancer in many foods such as canned tuna, dried soup mixes, canned vegetables, and processed meats.

Since it is difficult to avoid MSG and the other glutamates completely, it is best to treat for them if you are allergic. I have had excellent results in treating for sensitivities to MSG and other glutamates.

Gums, such as acacia, karaya, xanthan, and tragacanth gums, are another kind of additive that can cause problems. They are found in many foods, including yogurt, candy bars, cottage cheese, soft drinks, soy sauce, barbecue sauce, packaged macaroni and cheese, and numerous ready-made foods.

Some other problematic additives are benzoic acid, which is a food preservative; dipthenyl, which is a preservative for oranges; and hex-amethylenetetramine, a preservative found in canned fruit. Sodium pyrophosphoricum gives a red color to meat, especially processed meats. Sodium phenolphenolates, sodium sulfurosum, sorbic acid, urethanum (used in wine manufacturing), and carbamide (which is used to inhibit sprouting in potatoes) may all produce reactions.

Food coloring is another additive that can trigger numerous reactions in sensitive individuals. Many candies, such as jellybeans and hard candies, contain large amounts of coloring. Even foods sold in natural food stores may contain coloring, so beware. Reactions to food coloring can be serious, ranging from a severe constriction of the air passageways to coughing, runny nose, fever, hives, migraines, hyperactivity, insomnia, depression, and attention deficit disorder.

Pesticides can also be considered a food additive. They are particularly distressing because they are everywhere. Pesticide reactions can cause headaches, arthritis, breast pain, skin reactions, depression, hyperactivity, and irritability. Pesticides are difficult to get rid of once they are in the environment; even pesticides banned many years ago, such as DDT, still exist as residues in the soil and in people's bodies.

I remember treating John, age fifty, who was HIV-positive and suffered from severe fatigue and depression. One of the breakthroughs in our treatment occurred when I treated him for pesticides, to which he was highly allergic. He told me that he had grown up on a farm and helped his father spray the plants and trees with pesticides.

Of course, we should always eat foods that are free of pesticides, but they are so pervasive in the environment that they are very difficult to avoid. For this purpose, clearing an allergic reaction to these substances can be helpful.

ALCOHOL

Alcoholic beverages such as beer, wine, and liquor cause disturbances for many people. Treating for sugars and phenolics can usually clear an allergy to alcohol. Our clinic has successfully treated several alcoholics for their addiction to alcohol. With the help of other therapies as well, they have recovered. Often the craving for alcohol is really a craving for sugar. An alcohol allergy can weaken the bones by reducing the body's ability to make new bone to replace normal losses. It can also cause insomnia, arthritis, headaches, depression, kidney stones, candida infections, bloating, and asthma.

WATER

Surprisingly enough, some people react to their drinking water. One woman told me that she thought she was allergic to the bottled spring-water she used. Every time she drank it, she coughed. When I tested her, I found that she was indeed allergic to it. When she stopped drinking the water, her cough went away and her mucus production diminished significantly. Most people who have water allergies seem to be allergic to tap water; fewer have reactions to bottled water. Treating for your own tap water is something I recommend for those with asthma, severe bloating, eczema, or hives.

BREAST MILK

When a mother brings her baby to me with an upset stomach, I always suspect that an allergy to breast milk might be the culprit. As a matter of fact, I consistently find one out of five babies to be sensitive to their mother's milk. Clearing this sensitivity with the BioSET™ allergy elimination technique always makes a significant change in the baby's disposition and eating and sleeping habits. This allergy might have originated in the mother's allergy to such foods as milk products; tomatoes; cruciferous vegetables such as broccoli, cauliflower, brussels sprouts, and cabbage; and chocolate. The solution is to treat the baby for the breast milk allergy, supplementing with a digestive enzyme. This clearly may need to be done several times, as the breast milk content varies with the mother's diet. This can be done by dissolving one half of a capsule in water and giving it to the infant, or even by placing the enzyme on the mother's breast. When this is done, the allergic reaction will be immediately eliminated.

• • •

As you can now appreciate, any food can be a potential allergen, causing devastation in your life. People who have suffered for years with food allergies ask themselves painful questions every day: "What can I safely eat? How can I avoid allergenic foods when I go into a restaurant or when I eat at someone's house? Why does this only happen to me and not to my spouse? Why am I overweight when my friend, who eats whatever she wants, is not?" I hear these questions in my clinic every day. But I never become discouraged, because I know that the food allergy cure can relieve these frustrations. You can begin this journey yourself, right now, learning how to test yourself and then eliminate these allergies forever.

4

Common Ailments and Their Origins in Foods

Asthma, Headaches and Migraines, Chronic Fatigue, Arthritis, Hyperactivity and Attention Deficit Disorder, Ear Infections, and Eczema and Hives

✎ BARBARA'S STORY

Barbara, a forty-year-old woman, was coughing so badly when she came to see me that my receptionist had to move her from the waiting room into another room so as not to disturb the other patients. Barbara told me that she had asthma and that for the past two years she had had repeated bouts of asthma-related bronchitis, for which she had taken many courses of antibiotics. As a result of all these antibiotics, she now suffered from chronic vaginal infections and bloating after eating most foods. Were food allergies at the root of Barbara's asthma?

I performed a complete meridian balancing and detoxification exam and an enzyme evaluation on Barbara. I found two significant problems. Barbara had a weak spleen, the organ important in the manufacturing of lymphocytes and antibodies in a healthy immune system, and a hypoactive adrenal gland, the principal gland that fights allergies and supplies us with energy. She also had some difficulty digesting fats and sugars. I prescribed an enzyme to help her digest those foods, and another enzyme to support her spleen and immune system in order to strengthen her body's defense against infections. I gave her other homeopathics for detoxification and support to her kidneys, facilitating cleansing and purification.

Allergy testing revealed that Barbara was allergic to many foods in her everyday diet, primarily dairy products, breads, fruits, and eggs. I immediately began to treat her with the BioSET™ allergy elimination protocol, including the Level 1 preliminary treatments for allergies to one's own blood, organs, glands, and immune factors. I also treated her for amino acids, minerals, several sugars, eggs, milk, vitamin C, and several fruits.

After having her allergies to foods and some other environmental allergens cleared, Barbara did extremely well. Her asthma and incessant coughing were no longer a problem, and her bloating and vaginal yeast infections disappeared as a result of no longer needing antibiotics. In fact, since Barbara's first visit to my office, she has not required *any* antibiotics. Now and then she visits me to occasionally review her enzyme regimen, but Barbara has not been ill since her first appointment three years ago.

Asthma is just one of the many disorders I have seen resulting from food allergies. This chapter will discuss BioSET™ for asthma. It will also discuss the treatment of many other common disorders that I have personally worked with over the last twenty-two years that have food allergies as their root cause. These include headaches and migraines, fatigue, arthritis, attention deficit hyperactivity disorder, ear infections, eczema, and hives. Yes, the foods we put into our mouths every day can result in conditions such as these. The cure of dozens of disorders through the treatment of food allergies has already had an overwhelmingly positive impact on thousands of patients whom I have treated with BioSET™. It will no doubt change your appreciation of the power of the foods you eat.

ASTHMA

Asthma is a respiratory condition that affects more than ten million Americans and is one of the leading causes of school and work absences. In severe cases asthma can be life-threatening for both children and adults.

Asthma is a respiratory condition in which the bronchial tubes are hypersensitive to irritants and hyperactive. During an asthma attack the muscles around the airways tighten, the linings become inflamed and swollen, and the glands produce an overabundance of thick mucus, further narrowing the airway passages. Breathing becomes difficult. This means that the body has less available oxygen and that carbon dioxide can build up to dangerous levels. Once an asthma attack has been triggered by some substance or condition, the airways in the lungs can become sensitive to other triggers, which results in chronic asthma.

RECOGNIZING AN ASTHMA SUFFERER

There are many different warning signs of asthma, and it is important for people to tune in to their own red flags. Most sufferers have one or more of the classic symptoms. The first is a wheezing and whistling that are heard when they breathe. The whistle can range from hardly noticeable to quite loud. The second symptom is coughing—a mild cough or a hack that just will not stop. The next classic symptom is chest tightness, like a tight grip around the torso. The last is shortness of breath. People with this symptom cannot take a deep breath. They feel as if they are trying to breathe through a straw, or worse, as if they are drowning. Breathing out is especially difficult.

EARLY STAGES OF ASTHMA

People who develop asthma often had eczema, which is an itchy skin condition, in early infancy. Eczema will usually affect an infant's cheeks and the creases in the elbows and knees of older children. Children with eczema are usually allergic to B vitamins (and foods such as yeast that contain high concentrations of B vitamins), vitamin C foods, such as all fruits and vegetables, and other food such as wheat and eggs. When these allergies are eliminated with the BioSET™ technique, the eczema usually clears up readily, and the occurrence of asthma later in life can be prevented.

However, asthma can develop at any age. About 25 percent of children with asthma develop symptoms in their first year. Asthma varies greatly from one person to another in terms of how severe the symptoms are and how often they occur. Most people, however, fit into one of four basic types: mild, moderate, severe, or coughing. Each type has particular treatment needs.

Fifty percent of asthma sufferers have the mild form and may have symptoms only once or twice a year. Because symptoms clear up quickly with the use of bronchodilators, most people with mild asthma use medications only when needed. Mild cases are most commonly triggered by viruses and viral allergies. However, food allergies are usually a fundamental cause, and treating them can help boost the immune system and prevent recurring viral infections that may trigger an attack.

Moderate asthmatics make up about 40 percent of asthmatics. They experience symptoms about once a month and may require daily preventative medications. For example, they may be prescribed inhaled corticosteroids as well as bronchodilators.

Five percent of the people with asthma are severe asthmatics. They require daily preventative medications, must use a bronchodilator as many as three or four times a day to maintain reasonable control over their condition, and are admitted to the hospital frequently. They experience wheezing and coughing most of the time, and find exercise and participating in sports difficult.

Coughing asthmatics sometimes complain only of a chronic cough that comes and goes. The cough tends to be dry and typically gets worse at night, and they may use asthma medications to control it. Coughing asthma is usually unrecognized as a type of asthma and is common in people of all ages. Some of these people develop the more typical symptoms of asthma later in life, and some do not.

Sara, age fifty-three, coughed every time she ate chocolate. Apparently she had eaten an excessive amount of chocolate when she was a child—all members of her family had, and she felt it was a family addiction. Chocolate is a common asthma trigger, along with coffee and other caffeine-containing foods. After I treated her with the BioSET™ allergy elimination technique for chocolate, her coughing nightmare ended.

Tommy, age four, came to see me with a chronic loose cough, which had started when he was age two and kept him up some nights. No medications were useful in reducing his symptoms. On their own his parents had figured out that his condition was related to food allergies, and came to me for treatment. When I treated Tommy for some food allergens, such as wheat, corn, bananas, peaches, and oranges, his coughing ceased and he no longer had trouble sleeping.

CONDITIONS RELATED TO ASTHMA

Chronic bronchitis and chronic sinusitis are respiratory diseases associated with asthma. I have found that asthma sufferers may experience bronchitis throughout the year, although it is more common for them to do so in the colder, wetter months when they are more vulnerable to infection. These infections may be linked with food allergies, or they may be caused by infectants that are allergens themselves. This means that when you eat a food, that food may very well have an allergic link with a bacterium that is otherwise suppressed by the immune system, causing it to surface. This explains the reactions of Elizabeth, a thirty-six-year-old asthmatic who experienced chronic bronchitis each time she binged on chocolate.

Allergic rhinitis produces an itchy and runny nose, sneezing, nasal congestion, and eyes that itch, tear, or are red. Some asthmatics have seasonal rhinitis caused by pollen in the spring, late summer, and early fall. Others have year-round rhinitis, which can lead to headaches and chronic congestion. Rhinitis is often related to foods such as milk, cheese, and yeast.

When the allergens are linked with bacteria or viruses, this condition can develop into chronic sinusitis as well as complications such as ear problems, diseases in the palantine or lingual tonsils, swollen adenoids, sleep disturbances, and otitis media. In children untreated ear problems may cause hearing problems later in life. Also, children with allergic nasal disease are often restless sleepers who wake up at night because of coughing, a stuffy or runny nose, and sneezing. They have a thick nasal discharge that is sometimes green. As the condition worsens they may suffer headaches and fever, eventually developing asthma or causing an existing asthma condition to worsen. Other complications of allergic rhinitis may include loss of taste and smell, resulting in decreased appetite and weight loss; oral or facial deformities; nosebleeds; and teeth grinding.

Up to 50 percent of all patients with asthma suffer from chronic sinusitis, which can aggravate an asthmatic condition and produce asthmatic episodes. The symptoms of sinusitis are headache and tenderness in the sinus areas as well as nasal congestion, postnasal drip, and stuffiness. The nasal congestion may worsen at night when the person is lying down, resulting in coughing. Other symptoms include pain and pressure in the teeth, cheeks, forehead, and behind the eyes; fever; sore throat; earaches; bad breath; and a decreased sense of smell.

✑ JONATHAN'S STORY

Jonathan, age thirty-six, came to me suffering from chronic allergy-related sinus headaches, which he had experienced his whole life. He had recently lost his sense of smell and taste, and he was subject to ongoing sinus infections, for which he continually used antibiotics. He also suffered depression due to his tiredness, irritability, and inability to breathe well or smell and taste adequately. For a period of eight months I treated Jonathan with BioSET™ for the many basic foods in his diet to which he was allergic, such as wheat, cheese, spices, yeast, bananas, oranges, and red food coloring. Gradually he regained his sense of taste and smell, and his sinus headaches and chronic infections disappeared. Life became better for Jonathan, and he prospered in his social and work environment.

Other lung conditions that can be caused by food allergies include emphysema and bronchiectasis. Emphysema is a disease characterized by the distension and damage of bronchioles and alveoli, breathlessness on exertion, and wheezing. Bronchiectasis is characterized by the dilation of the bronchi and the production of large amounts of sputum. Sufferers experience recurrent fevers and episodes of pneumonia. This condition may develop out of pneumonia or whooping cough. Both of these conditions benefit from food allergy treatments.

FOOD ALLERGIES ASSOCIATED WITH ASTHMA AND RELATED CONDITIONS

Foods or food ingredients may cause or exacerbate symptoms in those with asthma and asthma-related disorders. There are a few confirmed food triggers of asthma, such as milk, eggs, peanuts, tree nuts, soy, wheat, fish and shellfish, and sulfites in foods.

My research and clinical experience have confirmed these triggers of asthma, but I have found other offenders as well. These include seeds, citrus fruits, caffeine, spices, animal and vegetable fats, beans, yeast, alcohol, baking powder, baking soda, gums, and many other grains such as barley and rye.

Corn is another common food allergen. Some commercial adhesives, cornstarch-based powders, and even clothes starch can all provoke reactions in corn-sensitive patients. Just licking a stamp (with corn-based glue) can cause a reaction in an asthmatic who is allergic to corn.

Sulfites are particularly problematic, as they are used widely as preservatives (see page 48). Clearing sulfites may be a big help. But sulfites are also commonly used in the manufacture of many drugs, including asthma aerosols. This is dangerous, because if the person taking these drugs is allergic to sulfites, they may experience many side effects, ranging from restlessness to skin reactions, that may make the medication less effective.

HEADACHES AND MIGRAINES

Despite the anguish it causes, pain is an essential ally. Were it not for this warning signal, we wouldn't know when something was hurting us.

We tend to dismiss headaches, the most common type of pain and one with which we are all familiar, as a simple annoyance. However, like any other type of pain, headaches are the body's way of telling us something is wrong. Headaches aren't a disease. But they are a symptom of a larger health problem, one that needs to be investigated.

WHAT IS A HEADACHE?

The unpleasant experience of a headache comes from pain that is generated in the face, neck, scalp, and meninges, or casing of the brain. It only seems as though this pain is coming from deep inside your head; in fact, the brain itself does not feel pain. The illusion of pain inside the head is called referred pain, in which the brain misinterprets sensory input.

Referred pain is common. For example, when some people have heart attacks, they may experience the pain in their arms rather than around their hearts. The referred pain phenomenon, which can cause headache sufferers to sometimes mistake where the pain is coming from, can lead to misdiagnosis of the type of headache.

Jes Oleson, M.D., a neurologist at the University of Copenhagen in Denmark, suggests that headaches result from nerve stimulation in three different types of sites on and around the head: arteries and blood vessels surrounding the brain; muscles in and around the head and neck; and certain nerve cells, including those associated with the eyes, jaw, sinuses, ears, teeth, and spinal cord.

Characteristics of Headaches

Although each person experiences head pain differently, headaches can be classified according to the following characteristics:

- Sharp, shooting pains, which mean nerve problems
- Pulsating, throbbing, one-sided pain, caused by abnormal swelling and constricting of the blood vessels
- Dull, heavy, diffuse pain, caused by digestive disturbances, infections, or fevers

- Pressing, blinding, squeezing pain, indicating toxic overload, chronic fatigue, or emotional difficulties

Headaches As a Symptom of Other Conditions

Headaches felt in specific areas are often one symptom of a complex or group of associated symptoms.

- *Back of head (occipital region):* pelvic organ disease; digestive disorder or tooth infection; eyestrain; neck muscle pain; emotional tension; middle ear infection; adenoid infection; cerebellar tumor
- *Frontal:* digestive dysfunction; constipation; kidney disease; low blood iron (anemia); eyestrain; tooth infection; sinus infection
- *Side of head (temporal region):* a combination of pelvic and digestive dysfunction, or small-intestine disturbances; ear infection; tooth infection; disease affecting the tongue; brain disorder
- *Top of head (vertex):* disease in the ovaries, prostate, bladder, or uterus; anemia; nervous disorders; emotional strain
- *Eyeball region:* digestive or pelvic dysfunction; nasal diseases; eye inflammation
- *Upper jaw area:* dental pain (infections or amalgam poisoning); jaw problems
- *Lower jaw area:* dental pain (infections or amalgam poisoning); mumps
- *Total head:* toxic buildup; hormonal imbalance (particularly of the estrogen-progesterone ratio in women); liver dysfunction; bowel inflammation; emotional stress

TYPES OF HEADACHES RELATED TO FOOD ALLERGIES

Tension Headache

Tension headaches are very common. They begin as a dull, steady ache at the back of your head, then radiate around to the forehead and the temples. You feel as though a band is squeezing your head, making you close your eyes and reach for the bridge of your nose and then for a painkiller. You may also experience neck, scalp, or shoulder pain.

Tension headaches are so named because they are related to muscle tension. Most researchers think that muscle spasms, a clenched jaw, tight shoulders, or other tense muscles play a role in precipitating these headaches.

Sometimes a tension headache is the body's way of preparing for a fight, whether it is a struggle with a grizzly bear or a traffic jam. Your heart and mind race, your senses sharpen, and your muscles tense. The continual challenges of everyday life can cause muscles to become progressively tighter, culminating in a tension headache.

Cluster Headaches

Cluster headaches, though very rare, can be severe and debilitating. Once or twice a year they engulf the headache sufferer in recurrent waves that can continue for several weeks. They occur more often in men than in women and, unlike migraines, give no warning.

A cluster headache can last anywhere from fifteen minutes to three hours. The headache is concentrated on one side of the face—in the eye, the side of the head, and sometimes the neck. The headache sufferer's face may flush because of dilated blood vessels on the affected side. The eyes may tear, the nasal membranes may swell, and the nose may discharge watery mucus. Allergies have been known to precipitate cluster headache attacks.

Hypertension Headaches

Throbbing hypertension headaches usually start in the back of the head. They often begin in the morning or wake a person from sleep. Like migraines, they can also be accompanied by nausea or vomiting. Hypertension, or high blood pressure, causes these headaches, which may be related to an increase of blood pressure within the skull.

Rebound Headaches

Rebound headaches are throbbing, generalized headaches similar to migraines. These headaches are brought on by the overuse of analgesic medications such as aspirin and Tylenol and/or by a caffeine allergy. Even two aspirin and some caffeine on a given day can turn a mild headache into a debilitating one. I believe that some 50 to 80 percent of all those who suffer from frequent headaches are unknowing victims of rebound headaches.

TMJ or Dental Headaches

A temporomandibular joint (TMJ) headache is the result of jaw stress due to faulty bite, tooth infection, or other dental problems. A TMJ headache is usually described as a dull, steady pain on the top of the head that may be accompanied by jaw clicking and jaw pain. Although there is little evidence that links headaches to jaw or dental problems, the notion doesn't seem far-fetched. I have learned that food allergies sometimes cause TMJ headaches and related symptoms. Caffeine and sugar are the foods most likely to trigger these problems.

Exertion and Sex Headaches

Exertion headaches occur after aerobic activity, coughing and sneezing, sexual activity, or psychological stress. The pain is a sharp, throbbing ache either throughout the head or in one area of the head. I have observed that these headaches are sometimes caused by an allergy to foods high in lactic acid, the metabolite that accumulates in muscles when they contract. Lactic acid is found in foods such as milk and apples.

Headaches following sexual intercourse can be very severe and may be accompanied by radiating neck and upper back pain, similar to exertion headaches.

Sinus Headaches

Sinus pressure and sinusitis are the source of a dull, aching, intermittent pain that comes on gradually and is generally localized around the forehead or face, depending on which part of the sinus area is affected. Sinus headaches are usually associated with allergies, mainly to foods such as sugar, milk, yeast, and wheat. However, I have seen other foods involved. One of my clients who suffered from continuous, unrelenting sinus headaches became headache free after he was treated with BioSET™ for an allergy to beans.

MIGRAINES

The two main types of migraines are migraine without aura, sometimes called common migraine, and migraine with aura, sometimes called classic migraine. Migraine without aura is about twice as common as migraine with aura. The pain of migraines is intense and incapacitating.

Attacks of migraines without aura typically center on one side of the head. The throbbing, pulsating pain lasts anywhere from four to seventy-two hours. These headaches run the gamut from moderate to severe and are accompanied by nausea and/or intolerance to brightness and noise. Migraines without aura can be aggravated by routine physical activity.

Migraines with aura are headaches that develop over a five- to twenty-minute period and last less than sixty minutes. The sufferer sees a visual aura, which usually consists of bright, curved, jagged lines, but many other types of bright or colored figures can appear in the visual field. There may also be obscured or blurred vision in one eye. Numbness that spreads on one side of the face or into an upper limb is also a common symptom, along with mild temporary paralysis on one side of the body and speech disturbances.

FOOD ALLERGIES ASSOCIATED WITH HEADACHES AND MIGRAINES

When I first began treating headache sufferers for allergies, I had no idea foods could be the offender. But as one patient after another reported that their headaches improved after treatments for food allergies, I began to see a pattern. Delighted with these results, I decided to hold a seminar on headaches and their relationship to food allergies. Nearly one hundred headache and migraine sufferers showed up that evening. Some of them had conditions so severe that they lived every day of their life on prescription medication, and some had milder headaches that they relieved with the occasional use of over-the-counter remedies.

I spoke very honestly that evening about my allergy elimination work and my experience with treating headache and migraine sufferers. After forty-five minutes I opened up the floor for questions. I was astounded to hear most of these men and women name foods as their number one trigger of headaches. They knew firsthand what I had learned in my clinic over many years: What you put in your mouth each day can initiate those relentless headaches and migraines.

All alcoholic beverages, especially red wine and champagne, have been known to trigger headaches. Of course, a headache related to overindulgence is the most common, but for some people even a sip can be powerful. The great number of people who are allergic to red wine are often reacting to the high amount of tyramine and/or sulfites it contains. People who are allergic to beer are responding to the yeast and hops used in its brewing. Other alcoholic beverages that cause a high incidence of allergic reactions are vodka and port.

Black tea or green tea with caffeine are known to be headache initiators. This happens in part because of the expansion of blood vessels that is a rebound effect after the immediate vasoconstriction that occurs after drinking these teas. On the other hand, since the constriction of blood vessels is the *immediate* effect of caffeine, it is also used as a *remedy* for headaches and is therefore a common ingredient in headache pain relievers.

Salt can also precipitate headaches. Limiting one's salt intake often has little positive effect because salt is added to many foods, such as canned foods, chips, and even cookies, and is found naturally in others.

Since so many of us are allergic to calcium, lactose, and animal fats, cheese is an enormous insult to the brain and nervous system. Some other common foods likely to cause headaches are corn; milk; yogurt; nuts, especially cashews; soy products, such as soy sauce, tofu, tempeh, and tamari; wheat; and spices.

Other foods and substances known to cause headaches are food additives, including nitrates (foods high in nitrates include sausage, bologna, salami, pepperoni, hot dogs, ham, pork, Spam, organ meats, game meats, meat tenderizers, and fish such as sardines and herring); dried fruits with preservatives, such as benzoic acids; colorings, such as tartrazine; artificial sweeteners; overripe fruits; apples; citrus; certain types of fruit juices and fruits; members of the nightshade family, such as potatoes, tomatoes, and peppers; sourdough bread; doughnuts; and yeast.

❧ JUDY'S STORY

Judy, age thirty, came to me with symptoms including severe muscle aches, headaches, eczema, hives, and hay fever. Her main debilitating symptom, the headaches, was fairly new, having started only within the last three years. Judy had a very emotionally and physically demanding job as a lawyer with a big firm in San Francisco. She was beginning to miss days of work because of her headaches and muscle aches, and she was desperate to find a solution. Her physician had prescribed prednisone for her muscle aches, but this medication had caused a severe allergic reaction—hives, weakness, and swelling in the upper part of her body. Judy really did not know where to turn. One of the attorneys in her office, who was also my friend, referred her to me. He had once suffered from terrible headaches but was treated successfully at my office.

I performed a complete meridian balancing and detoxification and an enzyme evaluation examination on Judy. Both examinations revealed liver and kidney dysfunction and congestion, as well as protein, sugar, and starch intolerance, mineral deficiencies, and low adrenal activity. My recommendations for Judy included enzymes to help her properly digest the proteins and carbohydrates that she ate, enzymes for adrenal support, some mineral supplementation, and detoxifying homeopathic remedies for her liver and kidneys.

Next I performed a complete allergy test, which revealed that Judy was allergic to eggs, salt, cheese, yogurt, chocolate and caffeine, yeast, wheat, milk, nuts, and artificial sweeteners. I began to treat Judy for her food allergies with the BioSET™ allergy elimination technique.

Twenty-four hours later Judy called my office to report that she was experiencing a sense of well-being that she hadn't felt in a very long time. Her eczema had cleared up almost overnight, and her energy had shifted. She had been able to function at work that entire day without a noticeable drop in her energy level. We continued treating her remaining food allergies, such as wine, soy, food additives, corn, turkey, spices, and vinegar. Four months later, after the allergy treatments were repeated, I retested her. By this time she was experiencing very little muscle pain, her digestion was immensely better, and her headaches were few and far between. Aside from some environmental allergies, she was now completely allergy free. Judy's health had improved tremendously. She no longer had headaches, and most of the symptoms she had complained of when she first visited me were gone. Eight months later Judy wrote me a wonderful letter. She thanked me for her health and for "giving me my life back again," and said that she had gotten married and was very happy. She went on to say, "Dr. Cutler, you were the only doctor who approached my health not as a set of symptoms to be remedied, but as a whole body needing to be balanced and restored. And when that occurred, my health returned to me naturally."

✑ SHARON'S STORY

Sharon, a forty-six-year-old accountant, had multiple sclerosis (MS). Her most severe symptoms included migraine headaches and fatigue. She also experienced frequent bouts of numbness, fainting spells, dizziness, lower back pain, and heart palpitations. Sharon was aware that she had many food intolerances.

During her evaluation, I noted that she suffered from congestion and dysfunction related to her liver and gallbladder. Tenderness in the upper left quadrant of her torso indicated that she had some difficulty absorbing sugars. A slight kidney dysfunction was the reason for her low back pain. Many MS patients I have seen in my office over the years have concurrent low back pain, sciatica, and leg weakness. Sharon's history also listed digestive problems, including occasional gas and irregular bowel movements. A physical examination revealed that her abdomen was severely distended.

(continued)

I prescribed three enzyme formulas for Sharon, one for the digestion of proteins and sugars; an enzyme to help her body properly use calcium, magnesium, and trace minerals; and an enzyme to counter bloating and fermentation. I also gave her a detoxifying and drainage formula for her liver and kidneys.

I then tested her for food sensitivities. I discovered that she was allergic to animal and vegetable fats, wheat, yeast, coffee, caffeine, chocolate, beans, some alcoholic beverages, food additives including food coloring, fish, and all dairy products. After we cleared some of these foods and began her enzyme supplementation, her abdominal swelling diminished, her digestion improved remarkably, and her lower back pain was hardly noticeable. In fact, Sharon remarked that her spine had become more flexible since these allergy clearings. Added to that, she had not experienced a migraine since we had begun her treatment three months before. Although she still had periods of fatigue throughout the day, her overall stamina had begun to increase.

Sharon has been doing very well and is headache free. With the help of her enzymes and certain supplements, she can resist infections, work a full day, and eat pretty much whatever she wants.

CHRONIC FATIGUE

Most people who come to see me suffer from some form of fatigue, whether or not their condition officially meets the diagnostic criteria for the disease known as chronic fatigue immune dysfunction syndrome (CFIDS). While CFIDS is definitely more debilitating in its symptoms, any form of fatigue can be incapacitating, having an equally negative impact on one's life.

I believe most fatigue is the result of food allergies. This is most certainly true for CFIDS. In this chapter I will address the CFIDS sufferer, but all forms of fatigue can benefit from food allergy elimination.

Chronic fatigue is an elusive disease. The symptoms may come and go, or they may linger for years. The cause remains a mystery, although I believe it is rooted in allergies and chronic metabolic imbalances. Until recently the medical community as a whole was reluctant to diagnose chronic fatigue as a disease. When it first appeared, very few doctors would even regard it as a problem, while others sent their patients to a psychiatrist.

In 1984 the Centers for Disease Control finally developed a set of diagnostic criteria and gave this disease the name of chronic fatigue syndrome (also known as CFIDS). Outside the United States it's usually known as myalgic encephalomyelitis.

Chronic fatigue is a persistent combination of symptoms that include recurring sore throat, low-grade fever, lymph node swelling, headache, muscle and joint pain, emotional stress, intestinal discomfort, depression, and loss of concentration. Less common symptoms include severe premenstrual problems, stiffness, visual blurring, dizziness, nausea, dry eyes and mouth, chronic diarrhea, cough, lack of appetite, night sweats, sleep disturbances, irritableness, and forgetfulness. Patients often report that they came down with the flu and then never recovered. Fear may accompany the symptoms because they are so persistent and resistant to treatment. Most of the people I've seen with chronic fatigue syndrome say they were active, vibrant individuals until they suddenly got sick, often after a period of sustained stress at work. By the time they seek professional help, they're often so exhausted they can't get out of bed, can't concentrate, and feel depressed. This condition is frustrating for them and for their families.

It's not clear how many people suffer from the disease, in part because it is often unrecognized and unreported, but it is known to occur throughout the world. In the United States more than six million patient visits per year are made by people suffering from fatigue. But it is estimated that only two out of a thousand people meet the established criteria for a diagnosis of CFIDS.

Women are two to three times more likely to contract the disease than men, although the percentage of men being affected may be rising. The disease seems to be more prevalent among Caucasians and those who are well educated, although one study indicates that it is also widespread but underdiagnosed in lower-income and ethnic minority groups. In particular, airline personnel, hospital workers, and teachers have a disproportionate incidence of symptoms.

There are different levels of chronic fatigue, ranging from people who can function with some difficulty to those who are totally disabled. As previously noted, some people with CFIDS experience low-grade symptoms all the time, while others experience periodic episodes followed by remissions. Some are bedridden for months at a time. Approximately 25 percent of CFIDS patients are housebound, while others are able to function in a curtailed fashion. Most of the CFIDS patients I see, generally women, are between the ages of twenty-five and fifty. Many are being taken care of by someone else and cannot make their own meals or drive themselves. In fact, they are often just barely able to come in for their treatments. Typically, CFIDS sufferers tend to relapse after a marked increase in physical activity. Stress or mild exercise may exacerbate the symptoms, and changes in temperature, humidity, barometric pressure, and exposure to sunlight may cause a decline in functioning.

One characteristic of CFIDS that distinguishes it from normal fatigue is that adequate sleep affords no relief. In fact, CFIDS sufferers may sleep twelve hours or more each night and still be unable to function.

Depression is a common symptom of chronic fatigue, often brought on by the fatigue itself.

Sleep disorders are also common in chronic fatigue syndrome and can also cause chronic fatigue. Sufferers rarely wake up feeling rested. A person needs to achieve a certain amount of deep sleep each night in order to feel refreshed; otherwise she will experience daytime fatigue. Some CFIDS sufferers have insomnia, some sleep excessively, and others sleep only intermittently. If the sleep cycle is altered, it can contribute to ongoing health problems and can accentuate feelings of anxiety, depression, and fatigue.

Fibromyalgia, another immune disorder that is often confused with chronic fatigue, is characterized by pain in many areas of the body. The symptoms of fibromyalgia and CFIDS overlap considerably, with fatigue being the most debilitating. Other symptoms of fibromyalgia are gastro-intestinal problems, cognitive dysfunction, mood disorders, headaches, sleep disorders, sensitivity to cold, bloating, anxiety, and morning stiffness.

There is still no definitive test to diagnose chronic fatigue syndrome. Most people with CFIDS have normal blood tests, or if the test results are abnormal, they are not useful in making a proper diagnosis. Tests do exist that can rule out or eliminate other possible causes of chronic fatigue, which means that CFIDS remains a diagnosis of exclusion, rather than a diagnosis based on certain defining symptoms.

FOOD ALLERGIES ASSOCIATED WITH CHRONIC FATIGUE

In my experience, one of the chief causes of chronic fatigue syndrome is food allergies. Studies have found that 65 percent of people with CFIDS had food allergies or some other type of allergies prior to developing chronic fatigue. There is no one particular food allergy that is associated with all cases of chronic fatigue syndrome. Any food or foods may be the culprit. Usually people are allergic to the foods they eat most often, and will feel tired or depressed after eating a meal of their favorite foods. Other common symptoms include muscle and joint aches, poor concentration, and nervousness.

Many chronic fatigue syndrome patients report that their diet consists of carbohydrates, primarily rice, pasta, and cereals. These foods trigger the most common fatigue-related food allergies. Other foods linked to fatigue are wheat, corn, green peas, artichokes, carrots, and most fruits. Foods high in sugar are fatigue-producing. So if you experience mild or severe fatigue, you may find it quite beneficial to examine the foods you eat day in and day out and begin self-testing. I have no doubt you will see the connection that I have observed over many years.

∽∞ MARY'S STORY

Mary, a forty-five-year-old flight attendant suffering from chronic fatigue, came to see me complaining of unceasing tiredness, intermittent nausea, insomnia, and depression. After experiencing a bitter divorce, she noticed that her symptoms were becoming more extreme, and she was desperate for some relief. In her attempts to adequately support herself and her two children, she was not able to afford any time off work, but flying internationally was almost unbearable for her. She consequently lived on not much more than six or seven cups of coffee a day, sleeping pills, and antidepressants.

After taking a lengthy history and getting Mary's full dietary journal, I performed my customary evaluation. Her tests revealed liver, kidney, and lymph dysfunction, and poor digestion and assimilation of sugars. Other tests, such as blood and urine, revealed only slightly low levels of calcium. I recommended a sugar/starch digestive enzyme, a mineral/enzyme formula, an enzyme for adrenal support, and a liver detoxifier to be taken along with a lymph and kidney drainage remedy.

Allergy testing revealed that Mary was allergic to calcium; vitamins C, B_{12}, and B_2; cane sugar, glucose, sucrose, and fructose; and the foods she ate most often, such as coffee, chocolate, milk, wheat, corn, spices, and yeast. Other food allergies included food additives such as MSG, hydrolyzed vegetable protein, BHA, BHT, and food coloring; dairy, including cheese and yogurt; red and white wines; animal and vegetable fats; berries; and vinegar.

We began Mary's BioSET™ allergy elimination treatments immediately because her life was crumbling and she needed help fast. Mary responded quickly. Only two weeks into her therapy, she noticed her energy was increasing. She began exercising, reading, and scheduling more fun time with her children. I remember that even her attire seemed to change, becoming more attractive, and that she got a new stylish hairdo.

One month into her therapy, she told me, "Dr. Cutler, I am no longer plagued with that lingering fatigue and I feel radiantly healthy. Thank you so very much." Her brilliant smile brought tears to my eyes.

ARTHRITIS

Osteoarthritis is a degenerative disease affecting the joints. Cartilage lies between the surfaces of bones where they meet in a joint. Normally the cartilage provides a cushion between the bones, but the ability of the cartilage to repair itself does not keep up with the natural degeneration caused by everyday wear and tear. As the cartilage deteriorates, the ends of the bones grate on each other. This causes the ends of the bones to become enlarged and deformed. Deposits of calcium (bone spurs) collect, resulting in inflammation and swelling. These changes are believed to cause the pain associated with arthritis.

Arthritis is often associated with age, and most physicians consider these changes to be a normal result of aging. Osteoarthritis can occur in only one joint or eventually can involve virtually all joints of the body. Any joint can be affected, but those most often affected are the joints of the fingers and thumbs, neck and lower back, and hips and knees. Symptoms range from mild stiffness to crippling disability. The most common symptoms include stiffness in the early morning or following any period of rest, pain that worsens with joint use or increases with cold, and local tenderness and swelling of tissue surrounding the joint. Swelling and loss of adequate joint mobility are other common symptoms. Pain and inflammation, signaled by a warm feeling in the joint and redness of the skin around it, are the most debilitating symptoms and usually the first ones a person will notice. These symptoms often occur after movement or exercise, particularly toward the end of the day.

Osteoarthritis can also be caused by injury. Athletes frequently develop osteoarthritis in joints that they have injured repeatedly. Most football players, by the time they are in their mid-thirties, experience arthritis pain and discomfort. Joint instability, skeletal defects, and hormonal changes also play a role in arthritis.

Food allergies can play a huge role in osteoarthritis. Why is it that some people who have demonstrable signs of cartilage deterioration exhibit no pain or stiffness, while others are practically bedridden? Food allergies may be the deciding factor, and I have seen this evidenced in my practice countless numbers of times. I remember Sophie, a fifty-six-year-old woman crippled with hip pain as a result of arthritis. She came to see me six weeks before her scheduled hip replacement. I immediately prescribed a sugar-intolerant diet (see Chapter 11), since sugar aggravates arthritic pain and stiffness, and an enzyme to help her digest sugar and starch. I then treated her for several food allergies, including vitamin C and fruits, sugars, wheat, yeast, and dairy products. In ten days Sophie was pain free, and in two months she was 75 percent better. By the way, she canceled her surgery after the first ten days of treatment. Sophie is only one of many patients I have treated with BioSET™ who miraculously overcome the pain of arthritis.

FOOD ALLERGIES ASSOCIATED WITH ARTHRITIS

Foods that seem to exacerbate osteoarthritis are sugar, wheat, citrus, pork, eggs, and members of the nightshade family. Microorganisms such as bacteria and yeast can also trigger or aggravate the symptoms. These microorganisms are tied very closely with sugars in an allergic response. For example, consuming sugars can stimulate the growth of certain bacteria. Bacteria can cause autoimmune reactions in which the body attacks the tissues in which the bacteria lodge, thus creating inflammation and pain. These bacteria are usually cleared with the allergy treatment for sugar.

I have helped many arthritic patients to overcome their pain and disability, and in this book I will show you how to overcome these food allergies in the convenience of your own home.

ꝏ GRETA'S STORY

Greta, age seventy-six, was diagnosed with osteoarthritis eight years before she first came to see me in 1997. Greta felt stiff all over, most noticeably in her shoulders, knees, and hips, and she was having trouble getting out of bed.

For the past three years she had been taking several different anti-inflammatory medications, which gave her some relief. But as time went on she developed sensitivites to them as well as allergies to a number of foods, including dairy products, grains, and most fruits and spices. Among her symptoms were increasing joint pain, diarrhea, chronic sinus congestion, and hypoglycemia. Once a highly energetic woman, she was slowed down by the allergies and the arthritis.

A friend's daughter referred Greta to my office for food allergy relief, not in any way thinking that the allergy treatments would alleviate her arthritis symptoms. But Greta's life was about to change. An examination revealed severe bowel congestion, calcium deficiency, insufficiently active adrenal glands, and an inability to digest both simple sugars and complex carbohydrates. She also had pain and inflammation in her stomach area.

When I performed a complete allergy test, it revealed many food allergies. Among them were many minerals (including calcium and magnesium), dairy products, sugar, wheat, eggs, nuts, potatoes, tomatoes, and spices. Greta was also allergic to most vegetables, fruits, berries, alcohol, and members of the nightshade family (potatoes, tomatoes, eggplant, pimientos, and peppers).

I began treating Greta with BioSET™. Her disability prevented her from seeing me more than twice a month, but nevertheless she was committed to following through with the allergy therapy. Her first treatment was for minerals. When I treated her for calcium, it automatically cleared the sensitivity to most of the dairy products, and her shoulder and arm pain completely disappeared for the first time since 1988.

As a result of her treatment, Greta's stamina returned, and she was able to sleep all night without interruption. In addition, she could now take a calcium and magnesium supplement with enzymes, even though these minerals had previously irritated her stomach. It was one of the most dramatic and exciting improvements I had ever seen in a patient.

We continued to treat Greta for the rest of her allergies to the foods she most enjoyed eating, including grains, nuts, chocolate, and peanut butter. She also began taking an enzyme for digestion of sugars and complex carbohydrates and an enzyme to support her adrenal glands. Greta has not experienced any joint pain since her treatment for minerals. And she is a strong champion of home self-treatments for food allergies.

ATTENTION DEFICIT HYPERACTIVITY DISORDER

The official definition of attention deficit hyperactivity disorder (ADHD) as it appears in the *Diagnostic and Statistical Manual of Mental Disorders*, 4th edition, of the American Psychiatric Association includes a list of nine specific symptoms of inattention and nine symptoms of hyperactivity/impulsivity. Characteristics of ADHD typically arise in early childhood for most individuals. At this time, four subtypes of ADHD have been defined:

1. *ADHD—inattentive type* is diagnosed when an individual displays at least six of the following characteristics:
   - ❑ Fails to give close attention to details or makes careless mistakes
   - ❑ Has difficulty sustaining attention
   - ❑ Does not appear to listen
   - ❑ Struggles to follow through on instructions
   - ❑ Has difficulty with organization
   - ❑ Avoids or dislikes sustained mental effort
   - ❑ Often loses things necessary for tasks
   - ❑ Is easily distracted
   - ❑ Is forgetful in daily activities
2. *ADHD—hyperactive/impulsive type* is defined by an individual displaying of at least six of the following characteristics:
   - ❑ Fidgets with hands or feet or squirms in seat
   - ❑ Has difficulty remaining seated
   - ❑ Runs about or is excessively active (in adults this trait may be limited to subjective feelings of restlessness)
   - ❑ Has difficulty engaging in activities quietly
   - ❑ Acts as if driven by a motor
   - ❑ Talks excessively
   - ❑ Blurts out answers before questions have been completed
   - ❑ Has difficulty waiting in situations where people must take turns
   - ❑ Interrupts or intrudes upon others

3. *ADHD—combined type* is diagnosed when an individual meets both sets of criteria for the inattentive and hyperactive/impulsive types.

4. *ADHD—not otherwise specified* is defined by an individual who demonstrates some characteristics but has an insufficient number of symptoms to qualify for a full diagnosis. These symptoms, however, are serious enough to disrupt everyday life.

Children and adults who have ADHD exhibit degrees of inattention or hyperactivity/impulsivity that are abnormal for their ages. This can result in serious social problems, the impairment of family relationships, or lack of success at school, at work, or in other life endeavors.

Whether we call it hyperactivity, attention deficit disorder (ADD), or ADHD, this problem is being diagnosed more and more often among school-age children. Some experts estimate that as many as 3 to 5 percent of children in primary grades are taking Ritalin to control behavioral symptoms.

About 1 to 3 percent of the school-age population has the full ADHD syndrome, without the symptoms of other disorders. Another 5 to 10 percent of the school-age population have a diagnosis of partial ADHD, or a diagnosis of other problems, such as anxiety and depression.

Another 15 to 20 percent of children may show behaviors suggestive of ADHD, but a diagnosis of ADHD is not warranted if these behaviors occur only in specific situations, do not cause problems at home or at school, or are clearly identified as symptoms of other disorders.

Gender and age affect the frequency of ADHD diagnosis. Boys are about three times more likely than girls to have symptoms of ADHD. Symptoms of ADHD decrease with age, but symptoms of associated features and related disorders increase with age. Between 30 and 50 percent of affected children still manifest symptoms into adulthood.

CAUSES OF ADHD

Understandably, one of the first questions parents ask when they learn that their child has an attention disorder is "Why? What went wrong?"

Experts have investigated genetic and environmental causes for ADHD. Some children may inherit a biochemical condition that promotes ADHD symptoms. Other children may develop the condition due to abnormal fetal development, which has subtle effects on brain regions that control attention and movement. Researchers are finding more and more evidence that ADHD stems not from psychological factors or the home environment but from biological causes. Health professionals stress that since no one knows what causes ADHD, it doesn't help parents to search for possible reasons to blame themselves. It is far more important for the family to move forward in finding ways to get the right help. Scientists, however, do need to study causes in an effort to identify better ways to treat and perhaps someday prevent ADHD.

Recent research based on brain imaging has found that areas in the frontal lobe and basal ganglia of the brain tend to be reduced by about 10 percent in size and activity in ADHD children. Other investigations suggest that a neurotransmitter called dopamine may play a major role in ADHD.

Other research shows that attention disorders tend to run in families, so there are likely to be genetic influences. Children who have ADHD usually have at least one close relative who also has ADHD. And at least a third of all fathers who had ADHD in their youth have children who have ADHD. Even more convincing is that where one member of a pair of identical twins has the trait, the other twin usually does too.

HOW IS ADHD DIAGNOSED?

While there is no biological or psychological test that can make a definitive diagnosis of ADHD, a diagnosis can be made based on a clinical history of abnormality and impairment. An evaluation for ADHD will often include assessment of intellectual, academic, social, and emotional functioning.

Getting a medical examination is also important in order to rule out rare but possible causes of ADHD-like symptoms. Conditions and disorders producing symptoms that may mimic ADHD include reactions to medication, learning disabilities, hearing or visual impairment, behavioral or psychiatric disorders, and certain medical causes such as thyroid problems. Also, some very intelligent children who find themselves in an insufficiently stimulating environment may display ADHD-like behaviors. Children whose parents expect them to meet unrealistically high expectations occasionally show such behavior as well.

✆ JUSTIN'S STORY

Justin's parents brought him to my clinic two years ago. "Justin has always been underweight and small for his age," they told me. Justin was seven years old at the time, although his height and weight were that of a four-year-old. He was not a happy child and was very aggressive and hyperactive. Within the first half hour of his visit he scribbled on my walls with crayons, punched his mother in the face for no apparent reason, overturned a cabinet in my office, emptied his mother's purse and wallet all over my rug, and damaged one of my chiropractic tables.

When I feel overwhelmed and perplexed by a patient, I sit for a while and watch, listen, and try to feel what it would be like to be in their shoes. The only way I can really help is if I truly empathize with, instead of react to, an individual. So I asked myself, "What is Justin feeling, and what can I do to help?"

I asked Justin's parents what Justin ate every day. I was not surprised when they said, quite honestly, "Whatever he wants." His mother said, "Since Justin has always been small, and because he's very particular in his choice of foods, we allow him whatever he desires so that he will eat enough to grow. Practically every meal includes Chicken McNuggets from McDonald's, a milk shake, and maybe an apple as a snack. He also eats ice cream and cookies every day."

I suggested to Justin's parents that their son could literally be allergic to everything he was eating and that his behavior might be a result of this. Justin's evaluation revealed severe problems digesting sugar and starch, kidney and liver congestion, and a mineral deficiency. I gave Justin an enzyme to help him digest sugar and starch, a kidney detoxification preparation, and a liver drainage homeopathic remedy, as well as an enzyme for mineral absorption. Allergy testing revealed that he had allergies to yeast, sugar, vitamin C, fruits, chicken, minerals, wheat, and dairy—which covered most of the foods in his diet.

We then began BioSET™ allergy treatments. It was not easy to keep Justin still for more
(continued)

than a few minutes, but we were creative. I have a kids' room in my office filled with toys and music, and I brought videos into the treatment room for Justin to watch.

By the fifth treatment, a miracle had occurred. Justin walked into my office while I was sitting at my desk and gave me a flower. He then sat down purposefully and said very passionately, "I would like you to retest me after my last treatment. I think it worked." That treatment had been for sugars. He was right; the treatment had been successful. He then said, "I would like to do the next one."

I was so elated with his behavior that day that I impulsively hugged him. Justin was not thrilled with the hug but did offer a smile, which warmed my heart. I remember saying to myself, "He's totally different from the boy who first walked into my office."

Justin no longer suffered from ADHD following his first few treatments. His diet changed completely; it now includes vegetables, fish, and whole grains, and he rarely eats those Chicken McNuggets. Every once in a while I will see Justin's mother in town, and she always remarks on how I changed their lives. Jason is now almost ten and does very well in school.

FOOD ALLERGIES ASSOCIATED WITH ADHD

ADHD can be the result of almost any food allergy, but there are certain foods that seem especially likely to have that effect. These are wheat, dairy, corn products, yeast, chocolate, cinnamon, peanut butter, sulfites, food coloring, and MSG. ADHD is often associated with foods that contain salicylates; see Appendix 2 for a full list.

One of the substances that make up our nerves is phospholipids, which contain fatty acids. Some of these fatty acids, known as essential fatty acids, must be obtained in our diet because the body does not manufacture them. A lack of essential fatty acids, or an allergy to them or the foods containing them, may have an impact on the nerves and hence play some role in ADHD; indeed, levels of both fats and fatty acids tend to be lower in children with ADHD. Essential fatty acids can be obtained from foods such as fish, green leafy vegetables, flaxseed and flaxseed oil, walnuts, cashews, brazil nuts, almonds, pumpkin and sunflower seeds, some forms of algae, and evening primrose oil.

✑ MAX'S STORY: ANOTHER "HYPERACTIVE" CHILD

At the age of two, Max was unable to walk or talk. His behavior was erratic, aggressive, and sometimes violent. At times he would bite other children and scream for no apparent reason. At other times he was quiet, subdued, attentive, and friendly. His parents commented that they felt Max had two personalities and that something seemed to be triggering this abnormal behavior, even though they did not know what it was. They had gone to a pediatric neurologist for an evaluation, trying to find a cause for why Max could not walk, but they had not taken Max to any practitioners who specialized in behavioral issues. Max's parents had been referred to me by the neurologist.

I was never able to observe Max's more violent behaviors, but I did see that he was not walking, which was unusual for a child of his age. The neurologist had scheduled Max for further testing and diagnosis. But in the interim I tested him for food allergies and found that he was allergic to many foods, including milk, wheat, oats, chicken, corn, and chocolate. I was not sure what effects clearing these allergies would have on Max's present symptoms, but I felt strongly that we should do so before the neurologist's appointment, still three weeks away.

I began to treat Max with the BioSET™ allergy elimination technique. His treatments went well, but there were no dramatic changes in his symptoms, although his parents did mention that he had fewer outbreaks of aggression and tantrums.

Then one Wednesday afternoon when I was returning from lunch, my associate came up to me in the hallway and said, "Dr. Cutler, Max has begun to walk, and his behavioral problems are disappearing. His parents are thrilled, as you can imagine."

That was a profound moment for me. I realized that the extent of food allergies can barely be imagined, and that the results from clearing them are virtually unlimited. The importance of understanding the potential for health or illness that comes with each morsel of food we put into our mouth is overwhelming.

EAR INFECTIONS

Ear infections occur frequently in children between birth and age six. Nine out of ten children will have one or more infections per year.

Otitis media is an inflammation of the middle ear that may be caused by a viral or bacterial infection. An earache develops when the tissue lining the middle ear swells and the opening of the eustachian tube (which leads from the middle ear to the throat) gradually becomes obstructed; fluid may accumulate behind the eardrum, exerting pressure on both the eardrum and the sensitive structures that lie within and near the middle ear chamber. This can produce one of the most painful sensations a child will ever experience. Other symptoms commonly associated with otitis media include fever, drainage from the ear, sleeplessness, irritability, a change in eating habits, a change in hearing acuity, refusal to nurse on one side (for babies), and nasal obstruction or discharge. Middle ear fluid can also be present even when there are few symptoms. Chronic ear infections and fluid in the ear can lead to hearing loss and a delay in speech development in children.

The term "ear infection" is commonly used to describe problems associated with the buildup of fluid in the middle ear. In some cases bacteria are present and the use of the word *infection* is appropriate. However, many children with middle ear complaints suffer from mysterious inflammations that occur when no infection is present. Factors that may trigger ear inflammation include overtiredness, weather changes, water entering the ear (particularly from swimming), or strong emotions (especially if suppressed).

In the United States, ear infections accounted for 24.5 million visits to the doctor in 1990. Many of those visits resulted in a prescription for an antibiotic. Not all of those prescriptions were necessary for the children to get better, doctors now say. In fact, the overuse of antibiotics has had a serious side effect: the development of drug-resistant microbes worldwide. Resistant microbes mean that there is a real future possibility of outbreaks of bacterial diseases that no medicine can cure. Closer to home, taking several courses of antibiotics increases the chances that your own child will come down with an antibiotic-resistant bug. When researchers swab the throats or noses of kids who have recently taken a course of antibiotics, they are more likely to find drug-resistant bacteria lurking there.

Many physicians insert tubes in the ear for drainage, but this involves some risk of injury, as well as discomfort and inconvenience. As with antibiotics, this treatment is frequently unnecessary, because the problems of ear infections and fluid in the ear can often be eliminated by treating food allergies.

FOOD ALLERGIES ASSOCIATED WITH EAR INFECTIONS

Ear problems can be caused by allergies to foods. The allergic reaction can cause the tissue within the ear to swell, obstructing the eustachian tube and causing fluid to accumulate. The fluid may cause problems, or it may be invaded by bacteria.

Foods commonly associated with ear problems include milk products such as ice cream and foods high in refined sugars such as candy bars, doughnuts, and muffins. Other foods associated with ear problems are corn products, soy, peanut, eggs, yeast, and wheat. Oranges, tomatoes, and chicken are also sometimes problematic.

❧ GABRIELLE'S STORY

At age three my daughter, Gabrielle, developed a buildup of fluid in her ears. We noticed she was also experiencing some hearing loss. After many rounds of homeopathic remedies and herbal preparations, and a number of chiropractic manipulations, her condition was unchanged. I then brought Gabrielle to a local pediatrician who, after examining her ears, recommended that she have tubes inserted in them. After listening very patiently, I asked the pediatrician what she thought was the cause of this fluid buildup. She hesitated at first, but finally said that research suggested it was allergy-related. I acknowledged her diagnosis and told her I would consider her recommendations.

I knew that Gabrielle and I had some work to do. That evening I began to give her BioSET™ allergy elimination treatments. Within three months the fluid in her ear had disappeared and her hearing had improved. Gabrielle's most critical allergies were to soy, eggs, cantaloupe, grapes, apples, nuts, wheat, yeast, and spices. Another exciting improvement was Gabrielle's ability to breathe through her nose, something she had never been able to do adequately. Ten years later, Gabrielle remains allergy-free and is so healthy she participates on a championship team as a long-distance swimmer.

Many children who suffer from chronic infections or the accumulation of fluid can benefit from food allergy elimination. We don't need to remove all the foods they like from their diet. But when we eliminate their food allergies, their food desires will change and their health and well-being will be restored.

ECZEMA AND HIVES

Eczema, or atopic dermatitis, is a skin condition that can begin in infancy. In fact, 60 percent of children with eczema develop it before the age of one year. It tends to affect people with a family history of asthma, allergies, hay fever, or rhinitis.

Eczema has been described as the "itch that rashes." It is characterized by an intense itching that provokes scratching and keeps the skin chapped. Sometimes it oozes and can become infected. Chronic scratching can lead to dry, scaly, and thickened skin, a condition known as lichenification. Atopic dermatitis is thought to be caused by predisposition, environmental allergies, physical problems related to improper digestion, emotional difficulties and unexpressed strong feelings (a major factor after age), and liver toxicity. But medical science cannot pinpoint exact causes and can offer no significant treatment besides temporary relief of symptoms.

FOOD ALLERGIES ASSOCIATED WITH ECZEMA

What I have found, however, is that eczema is often caused by allergens, including foods. Treating for the appropriate allergen with BioSET™ can make atopic dermatitis disappear.

Milk, eggs, and peanuts are the most common offenders, but allergies to sugars, soy, wheat, citrus, fruit juices, food additives, sulfites, artificial colors, gums, tomatoes, meat, fish, pickles, relishes, vanilla, fats, and chocolate are also common.

HIVES

Hives, or urticaria, is another common skin condition that is frequently linked to food allergies. Hives is a skin disorder marked by raised, itchy red patches. Hives can appear very suddenly and may last for hours or even a whole day.

Foods commonly associated with hives are peanuts, eggs, shellfish, tomatoes, chocolate, nuts, spices, milk, food additives, artificial sweeteners, and prescription or over-the-counter drugs.

⊘⊘ PETER'S STORY

Peter, age four, came to my office with the most severe eczema I had ever seen. This little boy had no area of skin that was free of eczema patches. He scratched constantly—especially at night, which interrupted sleep for himself and his parents—and bled often. In an effort to avoid the overuse of corticosteroids, his parents had tried many natural, complementary therapies, but nothing had worked. In fact, with every treatment, Peter's condition worsened. His parents were desperate. They were able to see the relationship between foods and his condition and had consequently removed certain foods from his diet over the last two years. As a result, Peter's height and weight were far below the average for a four-year-old.

When I examined Peter, I found he had difficulty digesting most foods, so I recommended a chewable enzyme for general digestive purposes. Peter's parents mentioned that their son had experienced frequent loose stools since his birth, and they were concerned that he was not absorbing foods properly. His weight and height were obvious indications of this inadequacy. So we supplemented his diet with a digestive enzyme.

When I tested him for allergies, I found Peter highly allergic to almost all foods, which was not surprising considering his condition. I began BioSET™ allergy elimination treatments that day. Results were slow at first, but changes occurred abruptly when we treated Peter for vitamin C and fruits. After that visit, his sleep improved and his itching lessened. His progress was steady and consistent. Each time I tested the effectiveness of his last allergy clearing, Peter would show me areas of his skin that were now free of eczema. At this point he had been desensitized to milk, eggs, fruits, meat, chicken, turkey, spices, nuts, and rice. He was now eating much more and his weight had increased to a healthier level. He loved coming to my office and knew he was doing better. Everyone was sleeping better, and the whole family was happier and more energetic. We had come a long way, but we were only beginning.

(continued)

Although Peter continued to receive treatments at my clinic, I strongly recommended that his parents learn the allergy treatment themselves so that they could clear him at home for other foods and allergies.

Peter's mother recently brought me a picture of Peter at his last birthday. It was astonishing. Peter still has very small patches of eczema on his arms, but the rest of his body, face, scalp, and chest are completely clear and healthy.

❧ JACKY'S STORY

Jacky, age sixty-two, suffered from severe hives that she could usually control by avoiding the foods she knew were the culprits—turkey, spices, artificial sweeteners, food colorings, chocolate, aspirin, and yogurt. Recently, however, this strategy had not been working, and she was perplexed.

By the time I saw her, her condition had become very debilitating. Her feet and hands would swell with each outbreak, and the hives would last anywhere from a few hours up to two days. Upon testing Jacky, I discovered many more food allergies of which she was unaware. These included vanilla, onions, garlic, green beans, oats, avocadoes, gums, oranges, lemons, and berries. Not realizing that these food allergies could be eliminated, Jacky was relieved to discover which foods were triggering the hives, because she knew she could avoid them. When I told her that I could actually eliminate her problems, she was quite pleased. We began BioSET™ allergy elimination treatments, and within two months she was delighted to be free of hives.

She told many people about her treatments. When I was invited to speak on food allergies at our local bookstore, Jacky brought thirty friends and co-workers. The bookstore was packed. Jacky stood up in front of all these people and told her success story. She even mentioned that I had fixed the aspirin allergy she had suffered from her whole life. Eventually many of those people became my patients.

These case histories and success stories are only a fraction of the many that occur every day in my office. I am reminded of the old adage "You are what you eat." This is even truer when you are allergic to the foods that create your everyday aches, pains, and discomforts.

5

Complex Disorders and Their Origins in Foods

Depression, Digestion Problems, Weight Gain and Food Cravings, Infertility, Premenstrual Syndrome, and Problems of Menopause

The most effective treatments for any health problem are those that address the root cause of the condition rather than just the symptoms. Even with a good diet, those of us with food allergies are often malnourished, because we are unable to absorb nutrients from the foods to which we are allergic. These allergenic foods can be irritating to the intestine, further decreasing our ability to absorb them. And the extremely restricted diets often required by those with severe allergies may add to the problem of getting enough nourishment. In Chapter 4 you were introduced to the idea of the connection between food allergies and specific illnesses. This chapter continues the theme, examining a number of other disorders and problems that are frequently the result of the foods we eat.

DEPRESSION

Depression is an illness that affects a person's behavior, thoughts, and moods. Signs of depression include feelings of worthlessness, low self-esteem, perceived lack of happiness or gratification in life, perceived lack of reason for living, problems sleeping, early awakening, physical inactivity, lack of desire to socialize, and difficulty focusing and concentrating.

ॐ TED'S STORY

Ted, a twenty-five-year-old man, had dysthymia, a form of depression that is characterized by long-term symptoms that disrupt a person's performance. Ted was greatly troubled by his condition. Every two to three months he would experience a wave of depression that greatly undermined his well-being and quality of life. Almost immediately he would notice that his immune system was weakened and that he would come down with a virus or the flu. He experienced feelings of irritability, impatience, and fatigue that put a strain on his long-standing relationship with his girlfriend. At such times he didn't feel like exercising, which only enhanced his fatigue and poor outlook on life. His interest in his work would plummet and his performance would suffer.

Ted told me that he hoped a digestive and allergy evaluation and treatment would give him some kind of relief, because he had noticed some occasional digestive problems during his bouts with depression. I performed a complete evaluation and discovered that he suffered from liver congestion, an inability to digest protein and fats, and a moderate amount of food allergies. I immediately prescribed a liver detoxification remedy and enzymes to help him digest protein and fat, and I began BioSET™ allergy elimination treatments.

Ted was allergic to many foods, but what seemed very obvious from the start was his allergy to the amino acids taurine and phenylalanine. Many of the foods he ate often, including eggs, milk, beef, chicken, fish, soybeans, cottage cheese, baked beans, and bananas, were all high in these amino acids. After I completed Level 1, which included clearing his systemic allergies and boosting his immune system, I was able to clear Ted of his allergies to the amino acids.

Following these treatments, his food allergies were successfully eliminated, and so were his mood swings and depression.

Depression is the number one health concern that people research on the Internet. Interestingly enough, allergies are number two. Ironically, the two are interrelated. In my practice I have found that many types of depression can actually be cured or alleviated by clearing a person of their food allergies.

Depression is becoming more and more common in our society. Almost every woman I see in my clinic who suffers from fatigue also lives with depression. More than twenty million Americans, twice as many women as men, will suffer an episode of depression at some point in their life. In fact, depression is considered the number one mental health problem in the United States.

✐ KAREN'S STORY

Karen, age thirty-four, was referred to my office by a woman who works with recovering alcoholics, drug users, and overeaters. Karen suffered from chronic fatigue and also displayed severe depression with suicidal tendencies. She generally slept until one or two in the afternoon and was barely able to function. A psychiatrist had diagnosed her as having chemical imbalances and thyroid problems.

Karen had been taking antidepressants on and off for fifteen years, but they had ceased to be effective about a year and a half before I saw her. She had already consulted with a number of well-known physicians, psychiatrists, and psychologists, but so far no one had been able to alleviate her problems. She wondered if I could find a relationship between allergies and her fatigue and depression. During her first consultation she mentioned that as a little girl, she avoided many foods because they caused severe eczema.

Karen hoped that BioSET™ treatments might be beneficial. I had already had excellent results treating patients with mild depression and chronic fatigue, but her depression was more severe than any I had ever encountered. I viewed her case as a challenge and an opportunity to research the relationship between depression and allergies.

I began with an enzyme and nutritional assessment to determine which nutrients Karen was deficient in and which foods she could and could not tolerate. I saw that she had

(continued)

difficulty digesting fat, which is typical of people with thyroid problems. Consequently, I recommended a fat-intolerant diet (see Chapter 11). I also prescribed an enzyme to assist her digestion of proteins, sugars, starches, and especially fats.

Allergy testing revealed that she was allergic to all the B vitamins; sugars; minerals, including zinc, selenium, calcium, and magnesium; and most amino acids.

Karen was treated with the BioSET™ allergy elimination technique for these substances and came back reporting that she felt great for the first time in years. "I realize that this is how I *can* feel," she said. "I'm not as depressed or tired anymore." Unfortunately, this feeling did not last, but it did give her a glimpse of her true potential. Rather than getting discouraged, she felt happy that she now knew what it was like to be herself, and she was hopeful that she would be able to attain the same level of functioning again.

After reviewing some papers on depression and brain chemistry, I came up with some additional allergens that seemed to be related to depression. I treated her for essential fatty acids, soybeans, salmon, wheat gluten, alcohol, caffeine (she drank quite a bit of coffee), chocolate, and turkey. After these allergens had cleared, she noticed an enormous improvement in her energy level and in her behavior. We then cleared her remaining food allergies, which included spices, other grains, dairy, and fruits. At the end of three months, Karen's depression finally disappeared, and she was herself at last. She said she felt as though her depression had been surgically removed.

She returned several months later, after her treatments were finished, to report that her depression was no longer a problem and that she was optimistic about her health. She had begun to work and earn some money and consequently was feeling more self-confident.

Karen was one of the most difficult patients I have ever had, but also the most exciting and rewarding. I had always believed that while mild depression responds well to complementary medicine, severe depression does not. Mild depression is actually quite common. But severe depression can be frightening to deal with, especially when the patient is suicidal.

Treating Karen for food allergies to alleviate her depression was the key to our success. I can't say the same treatment would work for someone else who was depressed, but I do believe that allergy elimination is a promising and nontoxic alternative to antidepressant medication.

Depression is classified according to its severity and frequency of symptoms. *Major depression* interferes with daily activities such as working, sleeping, eating, and enjoying life. *Dysthymia,* or less-severe depression, is characterized by long-term symptoms that are not disabling but do prevent the individual from performing optimally. *Bipolar disorder,* also known as *manic-depression,* alternates episodes of depression with periods of mania, characterized by extreme feelings of self-confidence, high energy, and increased sexual drive. Bipolar individuals can change from a manic high to a depressed, frustrated, unhappy, irritable low in a matter of minutes. These mood swings may also occur over a period of months.

A tendency to depression can be genetically inherited, and it can affect people of all ages, from children to the elderly. Elderly people who experience depression usually show symptoms of insomnia, low energy, loss of memory, and weight loss. Depressed teenagers may become incommunicative and withdrawn and may experience physical symptoms, such as loss of appetite, headaches, fatigue, and bed-wetting.

Some women experience depression during their menopausal years, and this may be related to the drop in estrogen levels that occurs naturally at midlife. There are also psychological reasons for this state of mind. Middle-aged women are often caught between the demands of raising children and the responsibility of caring for aging or ill parents. Being tugged in so many directions—children, husband, parents, housework, job—often leaves these women little or no time for the self. Grief for the perceived loss of youth and fertility may be a factor, especially in American culture, which tends not to value older women as much as other cultures in which postmenopausal women are considered wise elders whose counsel and skills are much sought after. Food allergies may also play a role in depression around the time of menopause.

PSYCHOACTIVE DRUGS AND THE TREATMENT OF DEPRESSION

In our culture, depression, whatever the cause, is often treated with a variety of psychiatric drugs. Some psychiatrists and other mental health professionals are concerned about the emphasis on drug therapy for mental and emotional conditions. They worry that some medications are emotionally and physically addictive and/or may cause brain damage.

Prozac and other SSRI (selective serotonin reuptake inhibitor) antidepressants act by increasing the amount of the neurotransmitter serotonin floating around in the brain. However, there is concern that long-term use of SSRIs may cause the brain to quit producing normal levels of serotonin, resulting in depression when the drug is withdrawn.

Unfortunately, antidepressant drugs are still readily prescribed. I am always surprised at the number of patients who come to see me for a wide variety of chronic illnesses who have been prescribed antidepressant drugs for no other reason than that the drug "may help."

THE ALTERNATIVES TO PSYCHOACTIVE DRUGS

What are your alternatives? One, of course, is to examine your life and environment for situations and relationships that may be depleting your energy and joy for living, and work on making any necessary changes. Exercise is a second good tool for alleviating depression because it improves your mood, energy level, and performance. Clearing food allergies is another.

Clearing Allergies to Vitamins and Minerals

An allergy to vitamin B_{12} may lead to a deficiency in that substance, resulting in impaired mental function and depression, among other problems. Prolonged deficiency of vitamin B_{12} can result in permanent nervous system problems; this can occur in as little as several months.

One cause of a vitamin B_{12} deficiency is inadequate dietary intake. This is mainly a problem in people who eat a strict vegan diet, which includes no animal foods, and in alcoholics. Another cause involves the body's inability to absorb or use the vitamin properly. For example, when the cells of the stomach do not secrete adequate amounts of intrinsic factor, which is necessary for the body to adequately absorb B_{12} from the intestines, a deficiency can develop. Also, both hypothyroidism and hyperthyroidism can result in B_{12} deficiency, as can various intestinal conditions that cause malabsorption. Some drugs may interfere with the body's ability to utilize B_{12}, as do some parasitic infections and liver or kidney disease. An allergy to the vitamin may have the same effect.

I commonly encounter B_{12} allergies in my patients. After treatment, I see significant changes, especially in their mental clarity and the alleviation of depression. I will often supplement with a formula containing both vitamin B_{12} and enzymes (to allow for a more efficient absorption of the vitamin) for a period after the treatment. After two to three months this is often no longer necessary, since the ability to utilize the B_{12} in foods is then usually sufficient.

Other vitamins whose deficiencies are linked with depression and moods are folic acid, vitamin B_1, vitamin B_6, vitamin E, and vitamin C. Lack of zinc or magnesium is often associated with depression. Insufficient magnesium in the body can also cause anxiety, agitation, and panic attacks. (See Appendix 3 for a list of foods containing specific vitamins and minerals.)

I believe that depression can be a direct result of food allergies, but unfortunately this idea is not commonly acknowledged by doctors and psychiatrists who adhere to the standard medical model. If a person is allergic to amino acids, phenolics, vitamins, or minerals, ingesting these substances (or being unable to digest them) can directly affect his behavior and mood.

Clearing Allergies to Hormones

Another class of compounds that are of great importance in the full treatment of depression is hormones. Many different hormones are found in a variety of animal and vegetable products that we regularly ingest. These ever-present substances can cause depression if one is allergic to the hormone. For example, an allergy to sex hormones can account for menopausal depression, teenage depression, premenstrual syndrome, headaches, infertility, loss of libido, and hair loss. The common sex hormones to which I encounter allergies are estrogen, progesterone, and testosterone. Therefore, an allergy to any one of these substances can have extreme consequences for one's behavior and mood.

As odd as it might sound, I rarely encounter a female patient who is not allergic to her own sex hormones. Clearing these hormonal allergies can literally change a person's life. I see this all the time.

✑ TRISHA'S STORY

Trisha, a thirty-five-year-old designer, came to see me complaining of depression, adult acne, and migraines. She was desperate and suicidal. A psychiatrist had referred her to me for an evaluation for food allergies, hoping that treatment would help to alleviate her condition.

Trisha's history and diagnostic report from the other doctor revealed that she had allergies to beef, eggs, and lamb as well as to vegetable oils and dairy products. My testing confirmed similar results. I noted as well an inability to digest sugars, liver and kidney toxicity, and low adrenal function. I suspected that Trisha was allergic to her own hormones.

I explained to her what hormonal allergies were and how when one eats foods high in those hormones, they experience negative and powerful results. In many cases, we are not really allergic to those foods, but to the compounds found in those foods.

After consultation with her physician, I began treating Trisha with the BioSET™ system. I began with a liver and kidney detoxifier and drainage support, as well as a digestive enzyme for sugar and starch. After completing Level 1, we began work with Level 2, which includes the treatment of amino acids, phenolics, and hormones. We cleared her of estrogen and progesterone with the BioSET™ allergy elimination treatment. Within thirty-six hours Trisha felt her depression lift. She felt positive, energetic, and motivated. I was delighted.

Trisha is one of hundreds of women I have helped by clearing their allergies to their hormones. These allergies can ruin your life by causing marriage problems, child-rearing problems, low self-esteem, and severe depression. What is most disheartening is that you cannot escape hormones. Even though you may try not to eat foods that you know are high in hormones, pesticides have a hormonelike (specifically estrogenlike) effect on humans, and hormones have been found in food additives and our water supply, as well as in our own bodies.

Here is a list of the common hormones to which people are allergic, their corresponding symptoms, and the foods in which they are commonly found.

Allergies to *estrogen* can cause depression as well as dizziness, emotional instability, fibrocystic breast disease, a feeling of mental fuzziness, generalized itching, hormonal imbalance, hot flashes, infertility, irregular menstrual periods, manic-depressive illness, nervousness, premenstrual syndrome, postpartum psychosis, seizures, shakiness, sleepiness, spontaneous abortion, throbbing headache, vaginal burning, painful intercourse, and thinning of vaginal mucosa. Estrogen is found in animal protein, alfalfa, soybeans, legumes, anise or fennel, tomato juice, bruised and diseased carrots or potatoes, wheat germ, bran, peanut oil, and licorice. Phytoestrogens mimic the role of estrogen in the body, and they also bind to estrogen receptors that help control menopausal and premenstrual symptoms.

Allergy to *progesterone* can cause aching legs, backache, burning in the back of the head, pressure in the chest, depression, dysmenorrhea, fibrocystic breast disease, a feeling of mental fuzziness, gas, head pressure, headache, heart problems, hot flashes, itching scalp and hands, menstrual cramps or other problems, nausea, premenstrual syndrome, nervousness, sleep disorders, and weepiness. Progesterone is found in soy, wild yams, vegetable oils, beef, and cloves.

Testosterone can be responsible for acne, impotence, hirsutism, low sex drive, overaggressiveness in males, and sleep problems. Testosterone is found in animal products.

Clearing Allergies to Other Foods

Other food allergies that can cause depression are wheat, milk, sugar, additives such as MSG and aspartame, fermented foods such as sauerkraut, vinegar, caffeine, and yeast, and moldy cheeses such as blue cheese.

DIGESTIVE PROBLEMS

A huge number of people visit the drugstore every day searching for a remedy that will relieve their heartburn once and for all, cure their constipation or diarrhea, correct their bloating and gas, and stop their burping. These problems arise from an inability to digest foods, as described in Chapter 3, and from allergies to foods. The many digestive illnesses I have successfully treated are colitis, Crohn's disease, heartburn, constipation, diarrhea, and chronic bloating.

HEARTBURN AND GASTRITIS

Heartburn, commonly a symptom of acid reflux and gastritis, can be a precursor to an ulcer. An ulcer is an eroded spot in the lining of the stomach or the first part of the intestine, the duodenum. Some ulcers are caused by aspirin and other anti-inflammatory drugs. For many years doctors said that ulcers were not caused by bacteria, but in 1983 an Australian physician named Barry Marshall, working with colleagues at Royal Path Hospital in Australia, discovered that these doctors had been wrong. It is now known that ulcers are caused by a bacterial infection caused by *Helicobacter pylori*, which can be detected with blood, saliva, or breath tests.

Roughly half of older adults in the United States and Europe are infected with *H. pylori*. Those who are not and experience unrelenting heartburn or bloating immediately after eating are usually afflicted with allergies to foods such as fats, alcohol, chocolate, spices, peppermint, citrus, tomatoes, coffee, and calcium.

✐ BETTY'S STORY

Many years ago, a woman named Betty came to see me with symptoms of heartburn, severe bloating, swelling of her abdomen, and an inability to digest anything she ate. She also noted that over the previous two years she had experienced a chronic cough and periods of shortness of breath. At sixty-six, she was slim and healthy in every other way and was not taking any medication, which is unusual for a woman her age. In addition, her diet was impeccably well balanced, and she watched her intake of fat and sugar. Her complexion and her coloring were excellent. She walked a mile every day and did hatha yoga two or three times per week.

When I performed a complete enzyme and allergic examination, I discovered that she was allergic to calcium, coffee, chocolate, and tomatoes. Unfortunately, it turned out that Betty adored chocolate and could not let a day go by without having some. She had also mentioned that, based on a friend's recommendation, she had recently increased her calcium intake through both calcium supplements and dairy products, to help avoid osteoporosis.

I prescribed an enzyme specifically for acid reflux (see Appendix 1) and treated Betty with the BioSET™ allergy elimination technique for her allergies to various foods. Her chocolate craving ceased, her acid reflux healed, and she was very pleased.

IRRITABLE BOWEL SYNDROME

Irritable bowel syndrome, also called spastic colon, is a condition where the intestinal tract seems unable to function properly. Diarrhea and constipation may alternate, causing chronic bloating, gas, and painful cramping. About 15 to 20 percent of people in North America have irritable bowel syndrome. Food allergies responsible for irritable bowel include refined sugar; high-fiber foods such as brown rice; oats; high-fiber vegetables such as beans, peas, and lentils; and raw fruits, especially citrus, apples, grapes, raisins, cantaloupe, and bananas. Fatty foods, which can disrupt the normal movements of the digestive tract, are also implicated in this condition. Fatty foods include shellfish, potato chips, french fries, fried onion rings, and all vegetable and animal oils. Other foods include dairy products (more specifically the sugar lactose), wheat, coffee, and tea.

DIVERTICULITIS

Diverticuli are small pouches that form in the wall of the large intestine. When these pouches become inflamed and painful, the condition is known as diverticulitis. High-fiber diets can be extremely helpful for this condition—unless, of course, one is allergic to the many high-fiber foods recommended. In that case, these same foods can actually contribute to the cause of diverticulitis. Common allergens for those who suffer from diverticulitis include grains, legumes, vegetables, and fruits.

CROHN'S DISEASE AND ULCERATIVE COLITIS

Ulcerative colitis and Crohn's disease are two kinds of inflammatory bowel diseases (IBD) and are among the most severe digestive afflictions known to medicine. They can be difficult to tell apart, since both result in an irritated, inflamed bowel. The primary difference between the two diseases lies in their location in the body. Colitis affects the inner lining of the colon and rectum, whereas Crohn's can occur in any part of the gastrointestinal tract, but it most commonly affects the ileum, including the entire wall of the intestines. Once one of these conditions is diagnosed, the treatment generally recommended involves the long-term use of potent drugs and possibly major surgical procedures. Conventional medical authorities agree that there is no cure.

Crohn's and colitis are considered lifelong diseases. They may be inactive for extended periods of time, but periodically they become active again, with symptoms that might be worse than, better than, or the same as those of previous flare-ups.

The main symptoms experienced by patients with ulcerative colitis are:

- Fatigue
- Abdominal pain, especially right before a bowel movement
- Constipation
- Frequent passing of blood and mucus with stools

- Diarrhea in some cases, especially late in the disease
- Weight loss and loss of appetite
- Fever
- Possibly painful joints

The main symptoms of Crohn's disease are:

- Abdominal pain, often in the lower right quadrant, or bloating and gas
- Loss of weight caused by appetite reduction and improper absorption of nutrients
- Possible bowel obstruction, which may cause vomiting, pain, and distention of the abdomen
- Constipation and/or diarrhea, occasionally with blood
- Inflammation or ulceration around the anal area
- Fistulas, ulcers that tunnel through the bowel walls into adjacent tissues and organs, sometimes causing pockets of infection or abscesses
- Occasional leakage of stool into the urine
- Fever
- Persistent rectal bleeding, which can lead to anemia

Sometimes other areas of the body are affected by these bowel disorders, particularly the mouth, which may develop sores known as aphthous ulcers. On rare occasions patients may develop erythema nodosum, warm, red, tender lumps on the skin of the legs. Also, there is the possibility of arthritis-like joint pain and swelling, lower back pain or stiffening, and pain in the spine. Infrequently the inflammation may spread to the eyes, liver, or bile ducts. Children who are severely affected by the disease may experience a reduction in growth rate and delayed development.

I have been treating IBDs for almost twenty years with a success rate that is remarkable, given that these conditions are generally considered incurable.

❧ BILL'S STORY

A man named Bill in his late twenties came to see me complaining of severe abdominal pain, diarrhea, bloody stools, and weight loss. After diagnosing him with Crohn's disease, his doctor had prescribed steroids and told him to refrain from milk products. This last recommendation was helpful, but the long-term use of steroids posed enormous risks, and Bill's prognosis was not satisfactory. For that reason, he was referred to me for enzyme evaluation and allergy testing. After this procedure was completed, I discovered that Bill was intolerant of sugar and starch. I recommended he take a digestive enzyme before meals to improve sugar digestion. We then began treating him with the BioSET™ allergy elimination technique for Level 1 substances, followed by B vitamins, calcium, magnesium, and sugars. Since Bill began working with me three years ago, he has not had any serious exacerbation of his Crohn's, and he enjoys a varied diet.

Food allergies associated with irritable bowel disease may involve sugars, predominantly lactose, maltose, and glucose; minerals such as zinc and magnesium; and the bioflavonoid quercetin, which has been known to have a soothing effect on the intestinal wall once a person has been desensitized to it. Other food allergies associated with IBDs are wheat and other gluten-containing grains, including rye, barley, and oats; fiber, such as bran from oats or wheat; artificial sweeteners; dairy products, including milk, cheese, and yogurt; vegetables with a high sugar content, such as peas, carrots, and corn; nuts; fruits; beans; animal and vegetable oils; fatty acids; alcohol, wine, and beer; caffeinated beverages such as coffee and tea; chocolate and cocoa; carob; yeast; vinegar; food additives, including food colorings, modified vegetable starch, and sulfites; spices; and amino acids such as glutamine, which has been known to help heal the gastrointestinal tract after the allergy has been cleared.

❧ LEANNE'S STORY

A patient named Leanne, age thirty-three, came to see me for a number of symptoms, most specifically the chronic diarrhea that had plagued her for several years. She also suffered from bloating, was anemic, and had frequent outbreaks of acne. In addition, she noticed undigested food, mucus, and even blood in her stools. Certain other symptoms, including irritability, weakness, shakiness if a meal was missed, a need for coffee to provide energy, and periods of emotional instability, suggested that she also might suffer from hypoglycemia (low blood sugar).

On our first visit I did an exam that revealed a severe sugar intolerance, as well as congestion in the liver and kidney. Other laboratory tests performed indicated that Leanne's calcium and mineral absorption was lower than it should be, and that she had very acidic urine, indicating an overly acidic system.

I prescribed a mineral-enzyme supplement, a kidney- and liver-detoxifying homeopathic remedy, and a sugar/starch digestive enzyme, which would simultaneously assist with her acidic pH and her digestion.

I then proceeded to treat her with the BioSET™ allergy elimination technique for her Level 1 allergies and the following foods, which were found in her testing: B vitamins, sugars, chocolate, coffee, caffeine, milk products, gelatin, meat, lecithin, and wheat. When Leanne cleared caffeine, her coffee craving decreased, and she stopped drinking coffee altogether for the first time in ten years. She also began to have some normal bowel movements for the first time in two years, and her diarrhea became less frequent. Her acne cleared up by 50 percent, and her bloating diminished entirely and her stools became firm once she began taking enzymes and adhering to a sugar/starch-intolerant diet.

WEIGHT GAIN AND FOOD CRAVING

"I used to be a perfect size eight. I was so happy with myself! But then I started getting fat, and now I'm up to a size twelve. I exercised, but that didn't work, so I put myself on a diet. No change. After that I tried skipping lunch and breakfast. My friends keep telling me that eating only one meal a day is bad for me, and I know that. But I don't know how to lose weight, and I don't want liposuction. Sometimes I think I should plain starve myself. What should I do?"

Does this sound familiar? People of all ages, particularly women, are concerned about their weight. Some don't mind if they are ten or twenty pounds overweight. Others do care and try to follow a fairly good diet, one that is low in sugar and fat, but they still find those pounds creeping up on them. Some people go to the gym every day or hire a trainer and try to work off the extra inches, but still with no success. It can be very frustrating.

Unfortunately, in my experience, plastic surgery and diet medications are not the answer. And some medications used for weight loss cause additional medical problems, such as the heart and lung disorders developed by some people who took the popular phentermine/fenfluramine combination known as phen-fen. What a lot of Americans didn't know is that even before its FDA approval for weight control, European research had associated fenfluramine with brain damage in laboratory animals. Fenfluramine is off the market now, but some physicians still prescribe phentermine, an amphetamine, as an appetite suppressant. Many people do not realize that amphetamines, also known as "speed," are addictive. You can also build up tolerance to them. Any appetite suppressant effect ceases once the drug is discontinued.

Dieting and skipping meals are also ineffective as long-term weight-loss methods. About 95 percent of people who lose weight through dieting gain it back, and sometimes more, within a couple of years. Restricting one's food intake and skipping meals not only rob the body and mind of the fuel they need to operate at their best, but they ultimately backfire as a weight-loss strategy. Starving oneself—and dieting is perceived by the body as a state of at least semi-starvation—inevitably leads to either bingeing as the body takes over and tries to get adequate fuel, or wasting away with diseases such as anorexia nervosa, which can be fatal.

Anorexia nervosa, which affects mostly women, is an eating disorder in which a person restricts the amount of food she eats so much that she weighs 15 percent or more below her expected weight and often stops having menstrual periods. She restricts the amount of food she eats because she thinks that all or part of her body, such as her hips or stomach, is fat— even if she is not overweight. In addition to restricting the amount of food that they eat, people with anorexia nervosa may overexercise, often injuring their joints in the process, especially their knees.

About half of the people with anorexia nervosa also have another disorder called bulimia nervosa. Bulimia is an eating disorder that develops when a person, again usually female, has episodes in which she eats large amounts of food in a short period of time (binge eating) and then uses different methods, such as vomiting, to get rid of the food (purging). People with bulimia nervosa are usually very concerned about their body shape and their weight. In addition, they believe that they have little or no control over their eating behaviors, and often feel embarrassed or guilty about them.

As far as unwanted weight gain is concerned, I have found that digestive incompetence and food allergies are frequently the underlying culprits. And I've had enormous success helping clients to lose weight by establishing digestive adequacy and eliminating their food allergies.

We crave those foods to which we are allergic. That's a fact. I have found that the root of this addiction to the foods we crave is the body's allergy-related inability to absorb the necessary nutrient that is found in that food. Therefore, we crave those foods that are high in that nutrient. I remember a patient named Alyssa who craved orange juice and would drink four large glasses of juice a day. When I treated her for vitamin C and prescribed a vitamin C enzyme, her orange juice craving disappeared. As another example, doesn't everybody crave sugar? Ironically, a sugar craving is due to the almost universal allergy to sugar and to the equally common inability to digest sugar. When the digestion of sugar is restored and the allergy is eliminated, the sugar craving desists.

I have also had many chocoholics come to see me, and I mean *serious* chocoholics. Jane, one of my patients, was unable to walk near a candy shop without paying the store a visit. Unfortunately, she walked by a candy shop every lunchtime; you can guess what her lunchtime dessert was every day. Jane was concerned. Her weight and her cholesterol were going up, and so was her addiction. She noticed she needed more chocolate every week to satisfy her habit.

The reason a person craves chocolate is that it contains phenolics and amino acids, such as phenylalanine, tyramine, and caffeine. When the body is allergic to these substances, it can fiercely crave foods that have high amounts of these ingredients—therefore the chocolate frenzy. The addictive nature of caffeine and its ability to energize us and help us to focus also helps to explain our body's chocolate cravings. Of course, chocolate also has sugar in it, so there is more than one reason for our fixation.

Over the years I have seen numerous and sometimes very bizarre food cravings. I will never forget Lisa, a twenty-year-old college student who craved salt so badly that she would literally eat spoonfuls of it in between meals, and would always be munching on salty potato chips. Inevitably, her acne worsened, her feet swelled, and she was constantly thirsty, but yet she had to have that salt. I treated her for allergies to sodium and chloride with the BioSET™ allergy elimination technique, in combination with treatments for other minerals, and her salt addiction was alleviated.

Weight loss and food cravings can be treated successfully by establishing good digestion and treatment of food allergies with the BioSET™ allergy elimination technique. Then you can follow one of my diets, found in Chapter 11, with ease and lose weight successfully. Many times the weight falls off as soon as you begin taking a needed enzyme or soon after the Level 1 allergy treatments are begun.

You can discover the correct diet and enzyme supplements for yourself by answering the enzyme questionnaire in Chapter 10. Commonly, most people need the sugar/starch digestive enzyme and should be on the sugar-intolerant diet. This regimen will set you on your way for a stress-free life in which you are not tormented by weight problems and food cravings.

The most common allergenic foods related to weight problems are sugars; all grains, especially wheat, barley, and rye; all animal and vegetable fats; food additives, including food coloring; alcoholic beverages, including red wine, white wine, and beer; yeast; vegetables such as carrots, peas, potatoes, yams, and sweet potatoes; chocolate; and dairy products.

ᘒᕰ MAUREEN'S STORY

Maureen, a fifty-seven-year-old woman, was referred to my clinic by a psychologist for weight problems and sugar cravings. The psychologist felt that I needed to intervene in her case, believing that her addictive food-related behavior was a result of food allergies.

Maureen is one of the kindest people I have ever met, and I began to look forward to seeing her and treating her. She was seventy pounds overweight and consequently experienced severe hip and knee pain. She was fearful that she would eventually need hip and knee replacement if she didn't make some changes. That is why she had sought out the psychologist, because she had tried every diet available with no success at all. She was frustrated and yet needed an answer very soon.

I was excited to take on her case because I knew I could help her. I screened Maureen for any gross physical pathologies, ordering some blood and urine laboratory work to ensure that she did not have any physical conditions that needed further investigation. She had some history of low thyroid and was on thyroid medication. Her blood pressure was borderline high but seemingly under control and not yet a problem.

Her full examination and testing revealed liver and bowel congestion, an inability to digest sugars and starches, and a two-page list of food allergies. The only foods to which she was not allergic were oats and rice. I prescribed homeopathics for her liver and bowel, mineral-enzymes formulas, and enzymes for sugar/starch digestion and bowel regularity. I recommended that she follow my sugar-intolerant diet, and keep me updated on her progress. I also recommended that she follow an exercise routine of brisk walking for one mile three days a week. As soon as she began taking the enzymes and homeopathics, Maureen lost three pounds. She was ecstatic.

"It's only three pounds," I said, but she replied, "It's my beginning."

At that point we were ready to begin the BioSET™ allergy elimination treatment. After Level 1 was cleared, Maureen reported that her cravings, most notably for sugar, had less-

(continued)

ened. I then treated her for foods on her allergy list, which was greatly reduced after clearing Level 1. We cleared her allergies to grains, foods, oils, yeast, and sugars.

Each week Maureen came to the office, she reported weight loss. In fact, within three months, Maureen had lost twenty-five pounds. Once her allergy treatments were completed, Maureen was on her own, but she called periodically to report her continued success.

One day, when I hadn't heard from Maureen for a year, a new patient was brought into my office. When I walked into the waiting room, I saw Maureen sitting there with her sister, Cecily, who had come to see me for a consultation. Maureen was transformed. She was half her previous size and absolutely beautiful. And most thrilling, she was pain free for the first time in years. She told me she was convinced that her hip and knee pain had been a result of her food allergies. She had lost all the extra weight within seven months and has maintained her current weight with no effort at all. She is very committed to taking enzymes and staying on the diet. And her sugar cravings have vanished.

INFERTILITY

Infertility, or the inability to conceive, is becoming a vast problem, costing couples huge amounts of money as they explore ways to treat it.

MALE INFERTILITY

Male infertility is related most often to a low sperm count. This condition may be caused by numerous factors, including an infection after puberty that was accompanied by a high fever, unrepaired undescended testicles, taking certain drugs, trauma to the testicles, or an exposure to large amounts of X rays.

For the most part, however, a low sperm count tends to be related to more easily reversible conditions:

- A long illness or a chronic infection that has lowered a man's general health. Poor diet, strenuous physical exercise, lack of exercise, too much smoking and drinking, being overweight, overwork, tension, and fatigue can have the same effect.

- Abnormal temperature regulation in the testicles, which function best at a temperature slightly lower than that of the rest of the body.
- The vessels along which the sperm travel in men could be blocked by inflammation, an infection, or varicosity in the area.

Another problem can be poor sperm motility, when sperm are unable to travel from the vagina through the fallopian tubes to fertilize the ovum. This condition tends to be related to some of the factors mentioned for low sperm count and may also be due to an enlargement of the prostate gland, as well as to an imbalance of male hormones in the body.

FEMALE INFERTILITY

Either one factor or a wide variety of complex, interrelated factors may be the cause here. Common problems include:

- Endocrine problems. Difficulties of the pituitary, thyroid, or adrenal glands, which together regulate the menstrual cycle, may cause a failure of ovulation. To establish whether you are ovulating at regular intervals, you can keep a record of your body temperature using a chart and a sensitive thermometer. Before ovulation, the basal temperature on waking will be a little below normal. After ovulation it should rise by one-half to one degree and stay the same for the next two weeks.
- Fallopian tube problems. The tubes could be narrowed or blocked due to an infection of the womb or other diseases such as salpingitis (inflammation of the fallopian tubes), endometriosis, or tuberculosis.
- Fibroids. Fibroids can cause miscarriage early on in pregnancy, or a difficult labor. The origin of fibroids is largely related to a hormonal imbalance caused by an excess of estrogen.
- Prolapse. A malpositioning of the uterus could lead to infertility. I have been able to successfully reposition a prolapsed uterus through a visceral manipulation.

● Cervical problems. Infection or excess mucus from an inflamed cervix can block sperm. Polyps (growths projecting from the cervix) may also prevent sperm from entering the uterus.

There are, in addition, some causes of infertility that are shared by both the man and the woman. There can be antibodies in either partner that destroy the sperm. BioSET™ allergy elimination treatments have been successful in treating this condition.

In many women who suffer from infertility, absolutely no physical problems can be found. There may be a slight hormonal imbalance or a poor state of health from faulty diet and fatigue, but these conditions do not represent significant causes. I have found that infertility is caused by food allergies in about one fourth of all patients who see me because they are having trouble conceiving. The most common are allergies to those foods that contain high amounts of hormones. Therefore in cases of infertility I place all the female hormones high on my list of substances for which to test. Other significant allergenic foods are yeast, dairy products, grains, fruits, parsley, dill, fennel, legumes, tomatoes, peanuts, licorice, high-retinol foods such as carrots, green vegetables, yellow vegetables, sweet potatoes, egg yolk, liver, kidney, halibut, salmon, mackerel, crab, oysters, swordfish, and fish liver oils.

✌️ CAROL'S STORY

Carol, thirty-nine years old, had been trying to get pregnant for four years, with no results. She had tried everything except in vitro fertilization, because she was still searching for a natural, noninvasive solution.

Originally Carol came to see me for treatment of her food allergies and her elimination and digestive problems. She had no inkling that a food allergy could be an underlying cause of her infertility. I hesitated to mention this to her, not wanting to raise any hopes, since she had been through countless emotional episodes with this ordeal. I therefore focused on stabilizing her digestive processes and eliminating her food allergies. I prescribed an enzyme to help with the digestion of fats and some homeopathics for liver detoxification, and began treating her with the BioSET™ allergy elimination technique. After her allergies to Level 1 substances were cleared, I treated her for the amino acids and phenolics, and then proceeded to clear her for her allergy to progesterone.

A couple of weeks later I began to treat Carol for her remaining food allergies, such as yeast, carrots, green vegetables, and alcohol. Her digestion was much improved. Her constant abdominal bloating was gone and she felt much better. Two months after completing her allergy treatments, Carol called our office to tell us that she was pregnant.

PREMENSTRUAL TENSION SYNDROME

A woman's menstrual cycle can be divided into two phases. The follicular phase lasts from the beginning of menstrual bleeding until the release of an egg (ovulation). The luteal phase lasts from the time ovulation ends until menstrual bleeding begins.

Premenstrual syndrome (PMS) consists of symptoms that appear shortly before a woman's menstrual period starts and disappear soon after bleeding begins. By definition, PMS occurs only in women who have monthly periods, the time in the menstrual cycle when bleeding occurs. Women who are not menstruating, such as pregnant women or women who have gone through menopause, do not have PMS.

PMS can be hard to diagnose because symptoms can vary so widely. Symptoms of PMS can also blend in with other symptoms, such as those of depression or other health problems.

Many women have mild discomfort related to menstruation, such as cramps and mild breast tenderness, during their periods. These symptoms are considered a normal part of the menstrual cycle. A diagnosis of PMS is reserved for symptoms that occur during the two weeks before a woman's period begins and that are severe enough to disrupt a woman's life.

More than 150 physical and psychological symptoms have been

attributed to PMS. Symptoms vary greatly from woman to woman. They can include physical changes, mood changes, pain, behavioral changes, and other problems. Some of the most common symptoms are listed below.

PHYSICAL CHANGES

- Breast swelling
- Bloating, water retention, weight gain
- Altered bowel habits
- Acne
- Nipple discharge

MOOD CHANGES

- Depression, sadness, hopelessness
- Anger, irritability
- Anxiety
- Major mood swings

PAIN

- Headaches or migraines
- Breast tenderness
- Aching muscles and joints

BEHAVIORAL CHANGES

- Aggression
- Decreased alertness, inability to concentrate
- Withdrawal from family and friends
- Decreased sexual desire

OTHER PROBLEMS

- Food cravings, especially for sweet or salty foods
- Sleep disturbances
- Fatigue, lack of energy

BIOSET™ TREATMENTS FOR PMS

It has been my experience that PMS is frequently produced by food allergies. Female hormones and foods in which they are found are the number one allergy to consider with all female disorders, and most certainly PMS. An allergy to estrogen usually causes bloating, weight gain, water retention, excess irritability, and anxiety. An estrogen allergy also causes histamine release, which promotes itching and skin problems; an increase in prostaglandins produces a tendency toward pain, redness, and swelling and a relative increase in cramping of the uterine muscles. A progesterone sensitivity usually causes decreased libido, depression, and fatigue. Other allergens associated with PMS include calcium, magnesium, vitamin E, B vitamins, animal fats, alcohol, sugars, caffeine, pesticides, meats, and dairy products.

THE IMPORTANCE OF DIET, EXERCISE, AND RELAXATION

There are other changes that a woman can make that will decrease her tendency to experience PMS. Dietary changes can help a great deal. Sodium causes the body to retain fluid, so you can avoid some bloating if you cut back on salty foods. Women with diets high in sugar, alcohol, and caffeine seem more likely to have PMS symptoms, so decrease your intake of these substances. Clearing the allergies to these foods does not afford you the luxury of overconsuming them. They still are not desirable foods, and eating them will cause predictable results. Allergy treatments will reduce your cravings for them, so eating them in moderation should not be a struggle. The sugar-intolerant diet found in Chapter 11 is one that I usually recommend for women suffering from PMS, unless another diet is indicated by your answers to the enzyme evaluation questionnaire.

If you want to avoid the symptoms of PMS, I suggest that you:

- Limit your intake of refined sugar, as it depletes B vitamins, magnesium, and chromium, and contributes to increased insulin secretion, resulting in hypoglycemia.

- Limit your consumption of salt (table salt as well as the salt in prepared foods) to under three grams per day.
- Limit alcohol to one ounce per day. Alcohol destroys B vitamins, magnesium, and chromium, and is a potent depressant.
- Limit your caffeine intake to no more than two cups of coffee per day, as caffeine intensifies anxiety and contributes to fibrocystic disease.
- Increase vegetables to 40 percent of your diet, with an emphasis on green leafy vegetables and legumes. These are high in fiber and B vitamins and release energy slowly.
- Potassium is beneficial in decreasing water retention, so increase the amount of potassium-rich foods in your diet, such as sunflower seeds, dates, figs, peaches, bananas, and tomatoes.
- Increase your intake of natural diuretics such as artichokes, asparagus, parsley, and watercress.

Consider developing a regular aerobic exercise routine. (Consult your doctor first.) In one study, PMS symptoms improved in women who walked thirty minutes a day, three to four times a week.

Any relaxation method that works for you, such as yoga, deep breathing, meditation, or tai chi, will help you to cope with PMS.

◌ SYLVIA'S STORY

Sylvia, age thirty-eight, came to see me at my office suffering from severe symptoms of PMS, which included severe cramping, swollen breasts, irritability, and depression prior to and during her period. She had tried many different healing approaches, such as chiropractic adjustment, massage, acupuncture, and acupressure. While these therapies had given her some relief, none of them was completely effective. Sylvia was taking antidepressants and birth control pills to control her symptoms.

She suspected that a hormone imbalance might be a factor in her condition, and her poor digestion, which manifested as heartburn, flatulence, and constipation, made her think that food allergies were involved.

I began with Sylvia by performing an in-depth enzyme examination and a complete allergy test. Her enzyme evaluation revealed that she had a sugar intolerance, calcium deficiency, severe bowel toxicity, and low adrenal function. I prescribed a sugar/starch digestive enzyme, a mineral-enzyme formula, a colon health enzyme, and an adrenal health enzyme product that is high in B vitamins and vitamin C. We discovered that Sylvia was allergic to many foods, including eggs, calcium and other minerals, vitamin C, sugars, salt, phenolics, estrogen, progesterone, chocolate, coffee, caffeine, yeast, alcohol, milk, wheat, and artificial sweeteners.

I treated her with the BioSET™ allergy elimination technique with great success, and Sylvia was relieved of her premenstrual symptoms immediately. Within two months she no longer needed to take any medications.

MENOPAUSE

By the end of this century, more women than ever before will be experiencing menopause. Menopause, which takes place for most women between the ages of forty-five and fifty-five, occurs when the amount of hormones in a woman's body, particularly estrogen, declines. It is a process that usually begins two to five years before the last menstrual period, and is completed when one full year has passed without a menstrual period.

Decreasing levels of estrogen cause many of the long-term health problems, such as heart disease and osteoporosis, that can occur after menopause. However, symptoms associated with declining hormone levels can occur before menstrual periods have ended. This period of declining hormones is called perimenopause. Perimenopause can last several years and is marked by irregular menstrual periods and symptoms such as hot flashes, vaginal dryness, and mood swings. A woman who no longer has menstrual periods is postmenopausal.

The Food Allergy Cure is not the appropriate arena for a lengthy discussion of hormonal or drug therapy for the menopausal female. That topic is far too complicated for the scope of this book. But BioSET™ can be an adjunct to therapy for the woman who is experiencing many pre-menopausal, menopausal, or postmenopausal symptoms. Clearing food allergies seems to reduce the frequency of hot flashes and increase calcium absorption, therefore reducing the risks of osteoporosis. With the BioSET™ system I have also been able to alleviate patient symptoms of insomnia, vaginal dryness, loss of libido, and even hair loss. (Allergy treatments are not a substitute for hormone replacement in those women for whom it might be indicated.)

The food allergies most commonly related to menopausal symptoms involve vitamin B_6, vitamin B_5, PABA, vitamin C, bioflavonoids, calcium and magnesium, estrogen, and progesterone. Other related food allergies involve soybeans, flaxseed, parsley, dill, fennel, dairy products, rice, wheat, salt, seaweed, beef, pork, chicken, salmon, flounder, tuna, crab, shrimp, barley, peanuts, sesame, dried apricots, avocadoes, dates, pecans, almonds, cashews, Brazil nuts, corn, sunflower seeds, rapeseed, alfalfa, lettuce, sweet potatoes, egg yolk, olive oil, and wheat germ.

✌️ NINA'S STORY

Nina, age fifty-two, had just recently stopped having periods and felt miserable. She was plagued with night sweats, insomnia, mood swings, and dry skin, and she dreaded getting older. She was desperate for help and did not know where to turn. She had tried to prepare for this time of her life by reading some material on menopause, but now that she was deep in the experience, she felt confused and muddled.

After testing, I discovered that Nina's digestion was in need of support, so I recommended a digestion health enzyme as well as an adrenal enzyme that is excellent for women, and a mineral-enzyme combination. When I tested her for various food allergies, I found that she had far more than I had suspected. Nina was allergic to her own female hormones and to many foods. We cleared her food allergies and hormonal allergies using the BioSET™ allergy elimination technique. Immediately after the hormones were cleared, she was free of her hot flashes and insomnia. She was thrilled and very grateful. Nina's other symptoms were relieved when I cleared her of her remaining food allergies.

6

Food Allergy Testing

ood allergy testing is highly con-
troversial. The constant debate in the health care community about
which methods are best leaves allergy sufferers baffled and wondering
where to turn for real answers. Should they believe traditional medical
tests that show them to be perfectly normal? Or should they listen to their
own bodies, which signal them with every meal that something is out of
balance?

Day after day patients describe their frustration to me. For example,
Michele, a twenty-nine-year-old accountant, brought to her first appointment with me the results of three previous allergy tests and her health
questionnaire. She was clearly confused and frustrated. "Dr. Cutler," she
said, "I feel tired every day, even though I get eight hours of sleep. I'm
overweight, I crave carbohydrates, I bloat after eating lunch and dinner, I
break out in a rash when I drink wine, and I cry three times a week for no
reason. My allergy tests say I'm allergic only to fish, but I know other foods
are causing these problems, because when I don't eat, I feel wonderful.
Sometimes I feel I should eat only a minimal amount of food permanently.

Perhaps this is a sacrifice I need to make. Can you help me? I'm desperate, and I can't live this way my whole life."

Fortunately for my patients, I understand their dilemma—because I was in the same predicament until I discovered a way to assess and treat my food allergies successfully. Most food allergy testing is not comprehensive and is therefore misleading.

✏ ED'S STORY

Ed, age fifty-two, came to see me from a small town in central California. Even though Ed suffered from chronic fatigue, he was motivated enough to drive three hours to his appointment every week. His fatigue, disorientation, and depression had become so bad that he had been housebound for a year and had been forced to sell his very successful real estate firm. During his initial interview he told me, "I was sleeping most of the day and felt as if I were in a fog."

The man who managed to get Ed out of bed and to my office was a dentist, a friend of a friend. When he heard about Ed's predicament, he contacted him to express his concern and to offer help. The dentist talked with Ed about food allergies and the possibility that his problem stemmed from reactions to many of the foods he was eating. Ed told him that he had been through a battery of allergy tests that said he was allergic only to corn, which he avoided with no change in his symptoms. This dentist picked up one of my previous books, *Winning the War Against Immune Disorders and Allergies*, and proceeded to read to Ed about the many possible food sensitivities that most traditional testing is not able to identify, and their relationship to chronic fatigue and other autoimmune disorders. He then offered to assess Ed's food allergies with the muscle-testing process described in my book.

Lo and behold, Ed was allergic to almost everything he was eating. It was mind-boggling and overwhelming, but it also reassured him that maybe there was hope for his condition. This kind friend then phoned me and asked if I could assist him in trying to treat Ed in a preliminary way with the BioSET™ allergy elimination technique. His hope was that this might at least give Ed enough relief so that he could get out of bed and come to my office for the remainder of his therapy. I agreed and instructed the dentist in the allergy elimination technique that I will also be teaching you.

The dentist and I spoke throughout the next two weeks about Ed's progress, and the reports were outstanding. After only one week of treatment, Ed was out of bed, having visitors, reading, and walking three blocks a day. I was so moved by this case that it inspired me to develop an allergy elimination technique that anyone can perform at home. Food allergy elimination saved Ed's life, and this case history paved the way for the future of BioSET™ at-home treatment.

Ed just recently visited my office after three years. Not only has he been well, but he has opened another real estate office that is even more successful than the first. Ed considers me his best friend.

HOW TRADITIONAL MEDICAL PRACTITIONERS TEST FOR ALLERGIES

In addition to self-assessment questionnaires to ascertain the probability of food allergies, there are a number of different allergy tests administered by qualified health professionals. These include skin reaction tests, blood tests, pulse tests, cytotoxic testing, antigen leukocyte cellular antibody testing (ALCAT), serial dilution endpoint titration, provocative neutralization testing, muscle tests, and electronic tests. Most of these testing procedures are incomplete and unreliable, but nonetheless they are still used and recognized in the allergy-testing domain. I describe them here to help the reader understand why traditional medical tests for allergies have not, and cannot, adequately diagnose the source of their allergies, and also to answer the questions you probably have after undergoing these tests.

SCRATCH TEST/SKIN REACTION TEST

Some tests for allergies involve provoking an allergic reaction on the skin by exposing it to a minute amount of an allergen. Most commonly this is accomplished by applying drops of an allergenic extract to a skin surface that has been pricked or scratched. Other possibilities include:

- Intradermal test: introducing a small quantity of allergenic extract between the layers of skin with a needle

- Patch test: placing a piece of gauze soaked in a suspected allergen over the skin for a prolonged period of time
- Conjunctival test (rarely used today): putting a drop of an allergenic extract in the eye

If a test is positive, the site of the exposure will swell and the surrounding area will become inflamed. This is generally not useful in determining food allergies. It is important to realize that the reason most people suffer reactions to foods that weren't detected with traditional testing is that those tests only evaluate specific types of reactions—yet allergies can be triggered by a number of different mechanisms. For example, conventional allergy tests that measure antibodies (the artillery of the immune system) measure just one particular type of antibody (IgE), which is only released in about 15 percent of food reactions. Also keep in mind that traditional allergy tests were designed primarily to detect sensitivities to inhalant allergens, which operate very differently in the body than food allergies.

Another drawback to these types of testing is that once a substance is introduced into the patient's system, a reaction may occur immediately within fifteen minutes, or it might be delayed and occur as much as fifteen hours later. Since I have seen this happen frequently in my practice, it is my opinion that depending on immediate skin reactions to testing can be misleading and generate a lot of false negatives.

BLOOD TEST (RAST)

The radio allergosorbent test (RAST) is an initial lab test done on a patient's blood sample to measure the number of IgE antibodies contained in it. The rationale behind it is that the number of antibodies increases with the severity of the patient's allergy, reflecting increased efforts by the immune system to protect against the allergen. The blood sample is tested for the specific IgE antibodies that the body would manufacture in the presence of the most likely allergens in the patient's environment. The drawbacks are that this test can be costly and that it could yield false results if a person has not eaten a particular food for several months. For example, over the years many perplexed patients have handed me the results of their RAST tests and asked me why foods that made them feel terrible weren't picked up. One patient remarked that she knew she felt sleepy after ingesting wheat, but that wheat was not considered an allergen on the basis of her RAST test. I was not surprised when she told me she had not eaten wheat during the nine months prior to the test. No antibodies will show up if a food has not been eaten for a few months.

Another drawback to the RAST test is that it recognizes allergens only when antibodies are present. It completely fails to identify problem substances such as barley and corn, for which there is no antigen-antibody response.

PULSE TEST

The pulse test can be a practical diagnostic tool. I remember one woman who visited my office for food allergy desensitization. She had been practicing pulse testing for five years, and her listing of basic foods to which she was allergic was indisputable. I was quite impressed.

The pulse test was discovered by Arthur F. Coca, M.D., an allergist and immunologist. Pulse testing for allergies involves measuring a person's heart rate before and after exposure to a suspected allergen and is an effective method for determining allergic reactions to foods. First, take your pulse when you awaken in the morning. Very lightly press two or three fingers of one hand over the artery on the inside of the wrist of the opposite hand, below the thumb. (Other areas where the pulse can be read are the temporal areas of the skull, the back of the knee at the crease, behind the ankle bone, the carotid artery in the neck, and the groin area between the pubic bone and the front of the hip.) You then count the beats you feel during exactly one minute and write down that number. The average number of beats is typically sixty to eighty per minute. A normal pulse should be even and forceful, beating at a regular rhythm with no delays, interruptions, or other irregularities. You take your pulse again immediately before you eat a food to which you suspect you are allergic, and then take it again thirty minutes and sixty minutes after eating that food. An abnormal increase in the pulse after thirty minutes presumably indicates an allergy—provided, that is, that you do not have an infection and have not recently exercised. I have also experienced a lowered pulse as a possible indicator for allergies. Some allergic individuals experience no change in their pulse whatsoever, no matter what they eat. But for others it can be a highly useful tool.

Unfortunately, if one eats several foods at a time, which of course we all do, it is hard to determine exactly which food is causing the allergic reaction. If you decide to experiment with pulse testing, I would advise eating only one food at a time and waiting at least two hours before eating another food. It is useful to avoid the foods you want to test for one week before testing.

CYTOTOXIC OR LEUKOCYTOTOXIC TEST

The cytotoxic test is another blood test for food allergy detection. White blood cells drawn from the patient are mixed with different foods. A food allergy is suspected when the white cells show some deterioration. This determination requires that a skilled person read the slides. When the white cells are not damaged, the food is not considered an allergen. This testing procedure, like the RAST test, is also expensive and can produce false negatives when the food being tested has not been eaten for several months.

ANTIGEN LEUKOCYTE CELLULAR ANTIBODY TESTING (ALCAT)

The ALCAT is a common food allergy test used by many physicians. The method requires the use of a mechanism known as a Coulter counter that counts and sizes white blood cells and platelets. A person's white blood cells and serum are incubated with a particular food. Changes in the size and number of white blood cells are calculated and indicate an allergy to a particular food.

SERIAL DILUTION ENDPOINT TITRATION

This test is similar to traditional skin testing but with some slight differences. The food antigens are diluted to several strengths, and testing begins with a weak dose injected under the skin. The lowest dilution that produces a 2 mm weal (swelling) is considered the endpoint or treatment dose. Practitioners who utilize this method of testing claim that this procedure can accurately indicate one's degree of sensitivity to a substance. However, results for food allergy testing are not completely accurate for the same reasons that the basic skin or scratch tests are not.

INTRADERMAL PROVOCATIVE NEUTRALIZATION TESTING

This method is similar to intradermal testing but varies in that the substance being tested must produce not only a weal but also symptoms of the allergy. These reactions are then neutralized with subsequent dilutions of the allergen. The premeasured relieving dosage of this allergen is then used therapeutically by the individual to treat the allergy. This principle is similar to that behind homeopathic medicines.

SUBLINGUAL (UNDER THE TONGUE) PROVOCATION

In this test, the practitioner mixes food extracts with glycerin and squirts them under the patient's tongue. The doctor then takes the person's pulse and compares any symptoms both before and after the test for significant changes. Over a series of several visits, dozens of foods can be tested. This testing procedure can be useful for children or people who hate needles. Intense symptoms can occur with this testing, which can be helpful for the accurate observation and identification of allergens. But, on the other hand, these kinds of reactions can be a dangerous risk for those who are severely allergic. This process of testing can also be time-consuming because only a few foods can be tested at one time.

BIOSET™ METHODS OF ALLERGY TESTING

BioSET™ methods have proven in clinical practice to be more conclusive and more accurate in the evaluation of food allergies. These noninvasive, advanced techniques utilize acupuncture and chiropractic techniques for the immediate assessment of an individual's allergies.

Bioenergetic testing encompasses any tool that evaluates disturbances in the electromagnetic pathways or energy systems of the body. Practitioners of bioenergetic medicine consider these blockages to be the origin of disease and therefore the cause of symptoms such as headaches, chest pains, swollen glands, or joint pain.

For example, a structural misalignment in the lower back that causes the muscles to spasm can cause blockages along the bladder meridian, which runs the length of the back along both sides of the spine. This can lead to incontinence or urinary frequency, among many other possible symptoms. An example of these kinds of blockages can be seen in a patient who visited my office with severe gastric complaints. She had sustained a leg injury in the area immediately below her kneecap not long before, and was having stomach problems because part of the stomach meridian runs along the outside of the knee.

Two bioenergetic tools that I employ in the BioSET™ system are the muscle test and computerized allergy testing. Muscle testing is the evaluative mechanism of choice for at-home testing. The computerized tool is a more advanced system for practitioners of BioSET™ who have training in acupuncture and bioenergetic medicine.

7

Muscle Testing

Also known as applied kinesiology, muscle testing was developed in 1964 by Dr. George Goodheart, a chiropractor, as a way of reading energetic blockages in the body. Applied kinesiology was initially used to correct structural imbalances caused by poorly functioning muscles. The main objective was to support chiropractic adjustments of the spine, pelvis, and other articulations.

Since its conception, many practitioners have found that other areas of dysfunction can be recognized via muscle testing. One of the major areas was discovered by practitioners who experimented with muscle tests to evaluate factors contributing to stress in the body, or interfering with the body's adaptability and proper function. They soon recognized that allergies, nutritional imbalances, and emotional issues were potent stressors on the body's energetic pathways and easily detectable by muscle testing.

Step-by-step instructions for using muscle testing to identify food allergies begin on page 164.

Muscle testing has proven to be a fast, noninvasive method for uncovering allergies, nutritional imbalances, the physical consequences of emotional issues, and structural misalignments in the body.

Muscle testing in allergy diagnostics identifies blocks in the patient's electromagnetic energy field when it comes into contact with an allergen. Muscle testing bypasses the conscious and subconscious minds, making it impossible for the patient to influence the results. When someone holds a suspected allergen in her hand, a strong muscle will weaken if she has an allergy to the substance. This muscle testing procedure works not only with foods but with all allergens.

Most practitioners who use muscle testing refer to the concept of a "strong" or "weak" muscle. The results of a test do not depend on whether the actual muscle is strong or weak, but on how the nervous system is responding. In other words, it is more accurate to think in terms of the behavior of the nervous system rather than the actual power of the muscle. Over the years, this technique has undergone alterations, which have allowed for increased accuracy and more easily reproducible outcomes.

ALLERGY TESTING

During testing, the patient generally sits or lies down and extends one arm at a 90-degree angle, palm down, fingers pointing forward. The other hand rests in the patient's lap with the palm facing upward, not touching anything initially. To establish the baseline strength of the testing muscle, also known as the indicator muscle, the practitioner touches the patient's hand just above the wrist and pushes downward while the patient resists by contracting the arm muscles. This gives the practitioner a baseline measurement of the patient's strength.

At this point, the actual testing begins. In the hand resting in their lap, the patient holds a food or vial containing substance for which an allergy test is desired. The practitioner again pushes against the patient's other arm while he or she resists. If the person is allergic to the substance, the indicator muscle will immediately and markedly weaken. Any weakness or dropping of the arm is a sign of an allergy.

One of the reasons why muscle testing is so useful is its safety. Unlike other types of allergy tests, the person does not need to ingest the food to create an obvious reaction. Usually just touching the food in a glass vial pulls an unconscious trigger that weakens the muscle if a person is allergic. An arm test that remains strong indicates no allergy. Another major advantage to this test is that it leaves little doubt as to whether or not someone is allergic to a substance. After experiencing this technique or practicing it on others, you will find that it quickly becomes apparent how a patient responds to substances to which she is allergic.

Again, muscle tests done in this manner do not evaluate the power of the muscle, but how the blockages in our energy fields affect muscle function. Muscle testing procedures can detect hidden and active allergies, thus alerting the allergy sufferer to those substances that should be avoided.

So even if you haven't eaten wheat for some time due to a suspected allergy, your muscle will weaken when you hold wheat in your hand, whereas other testing will more than likely miss the fact that you react to this food. That is precisely why I prefer this testing procedure over most others. This method of testing identifies all allergies to foods, whether they exhibit high or low antibody reactions in the blood.

Glass allergen vials are the preferable medium for containing the allergen during this type of test. Small samples of suspect foods can be placed into these vials, or even into everyday glass items such as wineglasses or baby food jars. Unfortunately, plastic is not a successful medium for testing.

I prepare the allergen reagents I utilize in my clinic ahead of time. They do not contain the actual substances but instead are energetic carriers of substance signatures made by various homeopathic suppliers. These vials are easier to use and cleaner than food samples and are reusable, making them more practical in my busy practice. Either energetic vials or the actual substances themselves are acceptable and effective for home use. Food vial kits are available for purchase; for more information, see Appendix 1.

SELF-TESTING USING THE O-RING METHOD

You can test yourself for allergies, if a tester is not available, by using another form of muscle testing. Make a circle by touching the tip of your little finger to the tip of your thumb on the same hand. Then, with the index finger of your other hand, try to separate your thumb and little finger; in other words, try to break the circle. In a strong test, your fingers will be virtually inseparable. In a weak test, the circle will be easily broken.

To perform self-testing for allergies, hold the vial with the potential allergen in the hand forming the original circle, with the three unoccupied fingers. Your fingertips should be touching the allergen vial. If the circle remains strong when you try to pry it apart, you are not allergic to the substance. If the fingers weaken and separate, you are allergic. This technique takes practice to learn, but it can be a survival tool for severely allergic individuals who wish to test foods before eating them.

As previously noted, there are certain physical conditions such as arthritis or carpal tunnel syndrome that can make this technique ineffective, but for most people, this test works very well. It is also a great way to practice developing your sensitivity for all muscle testing. If for any reason you find it difficult to test yourself, just treat without testing, because there is no harm in treating yourself for something that isn't an allergen. Muscle testing is a simple tool that can be utilized by anyone at almost any age and at any time. This simple test, combined with appropriate treatment, can change your life—or even save your life.

Consider the experience of my friend Marie, a severe asthmatic. One beautiful summer evening, Marie and I were walking through the streets of Chicago on our way to one of my book signings. We spotted some luscious-looking yellow cherries being sold by a street vendor, bought some, and ate a few.

Ten minutes later, as we entered the bookstore, Marie began to wheeze. While the audience looked on in awe, I used the BioSET™ muscle test to check Marie for the cherries we had just eaten. I placed two cherries in her left hand and applied pressure to her outstretched right arm.

Her arm weakened immediately, confirming my assumption that she was very allergic to the cherries. I treated her then and there for the cherries, using the BioSET™ allergy elimination technique, and her wheezing ceased as quickly as it had appeared. The BioSET™ muscle test and treatment may have saved her life. I know it can deeply affect the quality of your everyday existence.

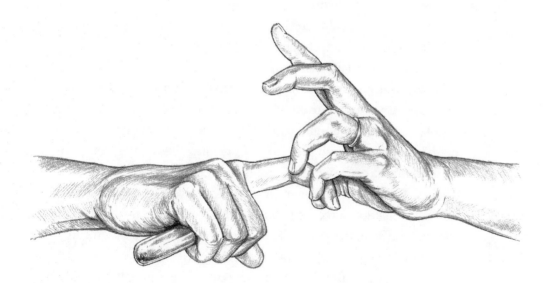

O-ring testing.

A TYPICAL VISIT TO MY OFFICE

A forty-six-year-old man named Bernard came to the clinic for examination and allergy testing. Bernard had suffered from food cravings, obesity, and depression for several months. He was referred to me by his wife, who received treatment of her chronic constipation and headaches with remarkable success.

When Bernard scheduled his first appointment, I sent him a tape and brochure on the BioSET™ system, an extensive questionnaire on his medical history, and an allergy and enzyme questionnaire for him to complete prior to his first visit. In preparation for his first appointment, I reviewed his health history and questionnaires. Bernard was instructed to fast for at least six hours before his first appointment (this is required for an extended enzyme evaluation), to drink only water during this period, and to avoid brushing his teeth or chewing gum before the visit.

When Bernard arrived at the office, I reviewed the questionnaire with him. A thorough survey of a patient's medical and family history is important during an initial exam. For example, factors such as a past illness, serious injuries, or familial tendencies toward diabetes or other disorders are highly relevant and are critical in helping me to interpret allergy test results and make enzyme recommendations accurately.

The first portion of the examination involves the meridian balancing and detoxification screening, during which we assess the areas of specific toxicity and weakness in particular organs. This examination can be carried out with muscle or computerized testing.

Bernard showed symptoms of stress in his liver, lymphatic, and kidney meridians, all frequent indicators of congestion in those body systems. Common symptoms linked to these systems include headaches, poor weight control, fatigue, and depression. Bernard was given homeopathic remedies for detoxification of his liver, and drainage remedies for his kidneys and lymphatic system.

The second portion of the visit is the fasting enzyme evaluation. When an individual is fasting, inflammations and enzyme deficiencies can more easily be identified. The areas tested are acupuncture meridian points and chiropractic reflex points related to organ and gland function. Stress in these areas can be observed when a patient experiences contraction or tightness upon palpation of certain acupressure points in the abdominal area. Some areas of stress noted during Bernard's examination related to the function of his adrenals, thyroid gland, gallbladder, and pancreas. I prescribed a number of enzyme formulations for removing organ stress, reducing inflammation, and improving function in these glands.

After the fasting enzyme evaluation, Bernard was given a drink that contained a broad spectrum of nutrients in a natural formula. Monitoring him after he drank it provided me with information on how well he was able to digest the different macronutrients: fats, sugars, starches, and protein. Bernard waited forty-five minutes while the drink moved through his system, and then we retested him with a regimen similar to the fasting evaluation.

The results of these two tests gave me a clear picture of how Bernard's body handled nutrients and what foods he had difficulty digesting. Based on this information, I recommended a specific diet that suited his needs. The test results showed clearly that Bernard was sugar- and starch-intolerant.

Bernard was given an enzyme formula focused on helping him with optimal digestion of sugars and starches, as well as enzymes for the support of his adrenals and colon health. I also prescribed digestive enzymes to relieve the stresses on his liver due to incomplete digestion. I explained that he would need to take the digestive enzymes before every meal, and the adrenal, colon, and liver enzymes between meals. (See Appendix 1 for a list of enzymes.)

I follow a very specific protocol for allergy testing and treatment. This protocol is the heart of the BioSET™ system, and it is the same one that I will describe in the home allergy testing sequence.

The first allergen to be tested is the blood. Many individuals are sensitive to immune factors in their own blood. It may be an issue of blood type or something related to individual chemistry. Under any circumstances, clearing the blood initially, and then using a vial with a drop of the patient's blood in subsequent treatments has proven to be a very important part of the BioSET™ allergy elimination technique.

We take a small blood sample from each patient and place it in a vial that we then use for every subsequent treatment in the BioSET™ process. The patient is muscle-tested while holding the blood vial in his hand. At later treatments, patients hold the blood vial and the other allergen vial and are treated holding both. I consider the blood vial as a way of customizing and individualizing each treatment for that particular person.

Regina, age forty-six, was one of the patients who helped me to pioneer this technique. Regina had always sensed that she had a wheat allergy. For example, when she ate a bagel, she would notice bloating and experience moderate intestinal cramping. But she loved bagels and found it hard to stay away from them. Therefore she was bloated most days. I treated Regina with BioSET™ for wheat, retested her, and found that her muscle test was strong. She was no longer allergic. At least, that was what I thought.

But Regina admitted to me that although she was much better, she continued to experience symptoms. I decided to muscle-test her for a wheat allergy while she was holding the wheat vial *and* a vial containing a drop of her own blood. Sure enough, she was still reactive. As an experiment, I then treated Regina for wheat again while she was holding both the vial containing wheat and the vial containing her blood. I asked her to eat a bagel the following day as a test and to let me know the outcome. Regina called me at noon the next day with great news. Not only had she been able to eat the bagel, she had also eaten some pizza and a sandwich with no bloating, cramping, or indigestion. She was elated.

Ever since, I have treated all of my patients with both the allergen and a vial containing their own blood. The results have been very successful. I have found that all of their food allergies have been cleared 100 percent when their blood was included in the treatment.

Again, it is not yet clear if it is the blood type or unique components of the individual's blood that facilitates the clearing of food, but for the purposes of home treatment, you can either make your own blood vial using a single drop of your blood, or purchase a homeopathic global blood vial (one suited for all individuals). This global blood vial has been proven effective for the at-home BioSET™ food allergy clearing. (See Appendix 1 to order empty vials or the homeopathic global blood vial.)

In Bernard's evaluation, his second round of testing was for allergic reactions to his organs and glands. It may seem strange that I do allergy testing for a patient's own organs and glands, but it has been my experience that a patient's sensitivity to his organs and glands can be a major obstacle to the effectiveness of therapy.

WHAT ARE ALLERGIES?

As I have noted, when we speak of allergy in the context of BioSET™, we use a somewhat larger definition than is commonly recognized by conventional medicine. Our definition of an allergy has been expanded to include everything from energetic blockage in the energy pathways of the body to observable allergies and sensitivities. In short, we include in our definition of allergy any factor that disrupts the body's energy system. No matter what type of disruption we find, the BioSET™ allergy elimination technque removes that blockage and restores inner balance. That is why testing most of the vital organs and glands is one of the first priorities in getting patients back to health.

Like most patients, Bernard tested positive for several of his own organs and glands. Treatment vials containing the magnetic imprints or signatures of his specific organ and gland sensitivities were prepared for use in later treatments in his program.

All of the BioSET™ allergy elimination treatments require a process of clearing through each organ and gland via the energy pathways (meridians) that supply them. If there is blockage, allergy, or dysfunction associated with an organ, often we are unable to completely clear the allergy until we also restore the balance in the organ systems. Otherwise the patient may experience treatment failures and increased sensitivity.

The third test we administer is a treatment for the immune system and its components. This includes white blood cells, immune mediators, antibodies, macrophages, lymphocytes, bone marrow, and lymph nodes.

Identifying and clearing blockage in the energetics of these cells and structures is essential to the success of BioSET™. Our bodies depend on the health of the immune system to fight diseases, infections, and allergies. If there is a sensitivity in one area, it can compromise the system as a whole, creating resistance and sometimes an inability to clear or desensitize allergies. After we isolated Bernard's specific immune sensitivities, another treatment vial was made for use in his therapy.

The fourth and final allergy test in the first level of the BioSET™ system is for digestive enzymes. These include amylase, protease, lipase, cellulase, maltase, and pepsin, among many others. Food allergies are often caused by poor digestion, which can result from insufficient enzymes due to poor diet, not chewing food sufficiently, or sensitivities to enzymes found in food and in the body. Clearing sensitivities to these enzymes with BioSET™ can be crucial in the treatment of many digestive disorders that must be taken care of before a person can live a life that is allergy free.

I always test these four categories with everyone—blood, organs and glands, immune factors, and enzymes. Only the items that show a positive response need to be treated. Some people may require treatment in only one area, while others may need treatment in all four. Specific items in each category can be tested and cleared together during the same treatment. These categories are treated individually on successive treatments.

I prefer clearing these four areas before treating for specific food allergies. I have found that taking care of them usually clears many food allergies automatically. Only after these categories are tested and treated individually do I then proceed to the next level of allergy testing.

In his first visit Bernard was tested for all four of these allergen groups. During the same visit, he was also tested for some very common allergenic foods, such as corn oil, milk, cheese, peanuts, walnuts, oats, wheat, citrus fruits, apples, food additives, chocolate, coffee, beans, and other foods to which he suspected he might have a reaction. I do this basic testing for the benefit of the patient who is just beginning treatment. In this way he can avoid the foods to which he shows a positive allergy response until we get around to clearing them. This avoidance can be instrumental in creating room for healing.

At the end of Bernard's visit, we reviewed our findings, including his detoxification and enzyme recommendations. I then scheduled him for four BioSET™ allergy elimination treatments. We also planned a follow-up visit for the next level of testing as soon as the first level has been treated and cleared.

Bioenergetic testing is truly unique in conventional medical circles. It tests on energetic levels as opposed to only the gross physical level. Allergies can be easily recognized on this energetic level, as well as toxins, deficiencies, and stressors. Energetic medicine opens up additional methods for discovering a deeper root to the many maladies physicians encounter in their practices, including chronic illnesses. It can also prove to be of vital importance in restoring overall health.

Food allergy elimination and restoration of health begins with testing foods to learn what you can eat and what foods disturb your system. Bioenergetic testing is at the forefront of accurate, comprehensive, and noninvasive testing. And, most significant, you can learn to perform self-tests so that you can begin your journey to freedom from food allergies, which is the purpose of this book.

Muscle testing is the first and most critical part of the BioSET™ allergy elimination technique. The gathering of accurate information is crucial in order to correctly evaluate and clear negative responses to allergenic foods.

Your body requires a certain amount of energy to keep its basic functions working. When you are healthy, these metabolic processes go on without your direct knowledge and everything is fine. When you eat something that is difficult for your body to handle, your system has to expend more energy to both keep you running and handle the stressful food. This pulls energy from the outer parts of the body inward toward the vital organs. While your body compensates for the stress, this creates a momentary weakness in the muscles of the arms and legs. This is the basis of the muscle testing technique used in the BioSET™ allergy elimination technique.

Based on this information, you can see that the explanation behind why muscle testing works is very simple. When your system is balanced, your energy is distributed evenly throughout your body and your muscles have what they need to easily and immediately compensate for stresses applied to them. You have the strength you need to respond when you need to lift a weight or move your body quickly. But when you experience stress—for example, if you eat a food that you're sensitive to—energy is pulled toward the interior of the body. Until your vital organs can compensate for the increased load, your muscles won't have as much ability to respond.

In muscle testing, we measure this strong/weak response. A strong muscle, when tested, produces a quick and forceful response when someone applies pressure against it. On the other hand, a weak muscle cannot forcefully resist even a small amount of pressure.

It is very important to remember that this strong/weak response test is not a measurement of how physically strong a person is. You are really determining what "strong" muscle control means for that individual, so that we can then observe what happens when you put him under stress and he goes "weak."

Naomi, a twenty-eight-year-old professional bodybuilder, came to see me for an interesting problem. In our first conversation she told me that whenever she ate chocolate before working out, her muscles would feel like putty by the time she got to the gym. She reported that her ability to lift was reduced by as much as 50 percent. After being treated for this allergy with the BioSET™ system, chocolate no longer had any negative effect on her weight training.

❧ DIRECTIONS FOR MUSCLE TESTING

For this type of testing, you will need a partner to muscle-test you if you are the subject. These directions are for the person performing the tests. First, gather the particular allergens you want to test and set them about four feet away from the person being tested. These can be either allergen vials or the actual food itself in a thin glass container, such as a wineglass. (Information for ordering food allergen vial kits can be found in Appendix 1.) Have the subject and the tester wash their hands prior to testing and between food tests. The subject should remove all jewelry, rings, and watches.

Before testing, have the subject drink a glass of water. This usually balances the electromagnetic energy of the body. Have the subject sit comfortably in a chair, feet uncrossed and flat on the floor. When testing the right arm, the tester should stand on the subject's left side; to test the left arm, stand on the right side.

- *Testing for the normal response.* Ask the subject to raise her right arm at a 90-degree angle to her body, palm down, fingers pointing forward, elbow straight. The tester should rest his right hand on the subject's left shoulder. With his left hand, he will make contact with the subject's right arm just above the wrist. The tester should then press the subject's right arm gently downward while asking the subject to resist against the downward pressure. (See illustration on page 166.)

  I find it helpful to begin each test by saying, "Resist against me" or "Don't let me push your arm down," to let the subject know that I am about to apply pressure. After a few tries I usually find that my subject and I will slip into sync, and then all I have to say is something like "Resist" each time I begin a test.

  Make sure to test only when the subject's arm is tense or very tight, not before. This helps to prevent false positives, which are weak muscle tests produced by some inconsistency in the testing.

  As you practice, you will notice that in a strong test, the subject's arm tends to lock immediately upon pressure from the tester, without the need for a great deal of force on either person's part. The muscle will have no give at all. During the initial testing this is called the baseline muscle response test. It represents the "strong" reference point from which you will test foods that you suspect weaken the subject's system.

- *Strengthening the response.* If you are unable to identify a strong muscle, a simple acupressure technique can usually assist you in this process. Stimulate two acupuncture points—CV17, located in the middle of the chest, and CV6, located below the umbilicus (belly button)—gently in a clockwise direction ten times simultaneously. Ninety-nine percent of the time a weak muscle will strengthen. If this is unsuccessful, contact a BioSET™ practitioner or treat the specific item regardless.

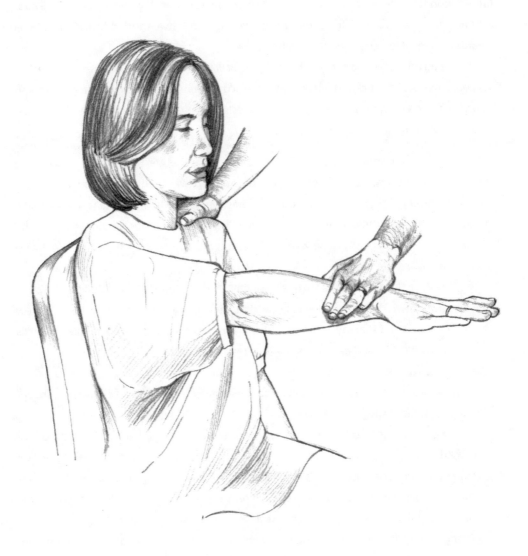

Muscle testing procedure.

- *Muscle testing for food allergies.* You are now ready to begin the food allergy testing. Place the glass vial or the particular food in the person's left hand, the hand opposite from the arm being tested. Make sure that the person holds the vial with his fingertips touching the allergen through the glass. Push down on the outstretched arm to see if the response is strong. If the person is allergic to this particular food, he will be unable to hold his arm firmly against your testing force and the arm will weaken or collapse. If the subject is not allergic to this particular food, his arm will not waver at all and his ability to lock against resistance will be evident. Any wavering is a sign of an allergy.

It is very important to remember that *you do not need to use great force when muscle testing.* To perform an effective muscle test, you need only to be able to feel a clear difference between the subject's strong and weak responses. When you ask the person to resist your downward pressure, you will notice an immediate locking of the arm (a strong test) or a weakening and collapse (a weak test).

You may then proceed to test up to ten items. The average person's arm will only be able to test about ten items at any one sitting before the arm will begin to tire. Over-testing can make testing inaccurate. You can double the number of tests by switching to the other arm.

Remember to have the person wash his or her hands in between items, placing a damp towel alongside your testing facility is recommended, and also remember to note the allergenic foods on a chart. I provide a blank chart that you can photocopy. These completed charts then become a guide for the treatments you are about to do.

TESTING CHART BASED ON THE BIOSET™ SYSTEM

Name of Substance	Passed	Not Passed	Additional Comments
Blood			
Organs			
Glands			
Immune system			
Enzymes			
Amino acids			
Phenolics and biochemicals			
Minerals			
Vitamin C			
B vitamins			
Sugars			
Vitamin A, vitamin E, and fatty acids			
Vitamin D			
Vitamin K			
Hormones (if needed)			
Additional Foods			

8

BioSET™ Home Treatment for Food Allergies

As you begin testing and treating your food allergies, keep in mind that the techniques I am describing are not designed to cure major illnesses; rather, they offer some basic tools for reducing and eliminating bothersome reactions to the things you eat every day. These methods aren't designed to substitute for appropriate supervised care by a qualified health care professional.

In order to begin the BioSET™ home food allergy treatment, you need:

1. A subject who wishes to receive allergy treatment. That subject can be you—instructions for self-testing and treatment are included in this chapter.
2. A quiet room away from any other activities that might distract from your treatment, such as ringing phones or children.
3. A sample (or vial) of the food that needs to be tested. You can use actual food or an allergen vial from an allergy test kit.
4. The step-by-step instructions for performing the home treatment,

which follow. A video is also available that serves as a guide to home treatment. (See Appendix 1 for additional information.)

For best results, treat for one food at a time. Often it is tempting to combine foods to speed up the treatment process, but my experience has taught me that the body responds much more completely to substances when they are treated one at a time.

STEP 1: SELECTING THE FOOD OR TEST VIAL FOR TREATMENT

At this point it is necessary to determine the order in which the allergies will be treated. Although BioSET™ home treatment is an ideal way to treat individual foods, it is most effective to treat allergies according to the basic sequence in Levels 1 and 2. Clearing these two groups of allergens will take care of the majority of common problem foods. If you don't have the sample kit, just begin with the food items to which you suspect you are allergic.

LEVEL 1: BALANCING THE BODY
- Blood
- Organs
- Glands
- Immune system
- Enzymes

LEVEL 2: CLEARING FOODS
- Amino acids
- Phenolics and biochemicals
- Minerals
- Vitamin C
- B vitamins
- Sugars
- Vitamin A, vitamin E, and fatty acids
- Vitamin D

- Vitamin K
- Hormones (if needed)

You can make your own food sample vials using empty sterile glass vials. They should be composed of thin glass (the glass in a spice bottle, for example, is too thick). A wineglass or small glass cup can also be used to contain the allergen—the thinner the glass, the better. (See Appendix 1 for information on purchasing empty glass vials.)

You can also get samples of homeopathically prepared allergens, produced according to the standards of the Federal Homeopathic Pharmacopoeia of the United States. These vials are excellent for use in BioSET™ allergy elimination treatment. (Information for ordering a Food Allergy Kit of vials is found in Appendix 1.)

STEP 2: PREPARATION

Have the subject drink a glass of water to balance his or her energy (polarity). This ensures that your test results will be more reliable.

It is almost impossible to muscle-test children under five, but these treatments work wonderfully on them, so just skip to Step 1 and treat for suspected allergens. Since the treatment consists of gentle acupressure massage, the massage tends to be relaxing and restorative even if your selection of the allergen is not correct.

STEP 3. TESTING

Begin by testing the blood vial. You can use either a blood vial prepared with a single drop of your own blood, or a universal blood vial that can be ordered (see Appendix 1). Place the vial in the subject's hand, and test according to the instructions on page 167. If the subject tests strong with the blood vial in her hand, that means the blood is not a stressor, and you can move on to the next item. If the muscle tests weak, you need a BioSET™ allergy elimination treatment for blood allergens.

If you are using the allergen vials in the test kit, the next test is the organ vial. If you are testing for food allergies with food samples, simply choose a food item that causes difficulty for your subject. The clearing procedure is the same for all the foods, organs, glands, and any other substances that test as allergens.

Remember, a strong response means that no treatment is necessary, and a weak response means that the item is stressful and needs to be treated for. *Once the blood factors have been cleared, the blood vial should be included with every treatment that you do from then on.* This means that the person being treated holds the blood vial in her hand, along with the vial of the allergenic substance being cleared. The blood vial should be in the subject's hand for all the allergy treatments and testing.

STEP 4: THE BIOSET™ ALLERGY ELIMINATION TREATMENT

After you've confirmed that the treatment item produces a weak muscle response, leave the sample in the subject's hand. For example, if chocolate produces a weak muscle response, have the subject continue to hold it. Add the blood vial to the hand holding the chocolate and begin the treatment.

ACUPRESSURE TECHNIQUE FOR BIOSET™ TREATMENT

The BioSET™ treatment for food allergies involves two parts:

1. Acupressure gently applied to the back
2. A series of nineteen acupressure points on the arms and legs

PART 1: GENTLE ACUPRESSURE ON THE BACK

In Part 1, you will work on the subject's back, performing this gentle acupressure technique from the top of the neck to the base of the spine. Performing these techniques correctly requires no experience in bodywork and can be learned very quickly. The acupressure points are located on both sides of the spine, about an inch from the vertebrae. Work the points directly beside each vertebrae—twenty-three of the vertebrae can be felt along the back, so you will work the twenty-three pairs of points next to each of these spinal ridges (see the illustration on page 174). Remember to have the subject hold the vial with the allergen and the blood vial during the entire treatment. This series is performed four times—each time with the subject breathing in a different way:

1. Holding the breath (taking a deep breath periodically)
2. Exhaling
3. Panting
4. Breathing normally

The BioSET™ acupressure technique can be performed with thumbs, fingers, or knuckles, although I use thumbs in the following description. Use whatever method feels most comfortable for you. When stimulating each point, use light pressure and move your thumbs in a clockwise circular motion about three times. The actual number of times necessary for appropriate stimulation is not fixed, but in my experience, three repetitions on each point should be adequate for most people. If the acupressure creates any discomfort for your subject, lighten up on the pressure. The changes you are trying to make require very little stimulation.

All the points discussed in the treatment sequence should be done in the same way. When massaging the points parallel to the spine, use both thumbs to stimulate the points on either side simultaneously. This saves time, since you will be doing the four repetitions:

Stage 1: Holding the breath. Ask your subject to inhale and hold her breath while you stimulate the column of points, moving down the spine. If your subject needs to stop to take a breath, that's fine. Resume as soon as she has inhaled and is holding her breath again.

Stage 2: Exhaling. Ask your subject to breathe out and hold the exhaled breath while you stimulate the points.

Stage 3: Panting breath. Ask your subject to pant quickly while you stimulate the points. The panting should be as quick and vigorous as the

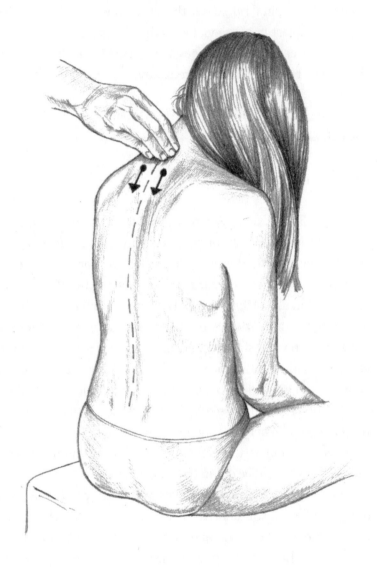

Treatment sequence. The subject can be fully clothed while receiving the acupressure. Massage the points from the neck to the waist area.

patient can manage. Asthmatics and patients with respiratory problems should do this carefully and only as much as they can manage. The treatment can still be effective even if the breathing pattern during this treatment is not perfect.

Stage 4: Breathing normally. Ask your subject to breathe normally while you stimulate the column of points.

Stage 5: Retest. With the sample still in your subject's hand, retest for the muscle response. If the treatment has succeeded, the muscle will test strong, indicating that the stressful response to the food has probably been eliminated. If your subject's response is weak, repeat the treatment.

When the testing and treatment have been performed correctly, the muscle will test strong after the first treatment about 90 percent of the time. However, the need for one or two repetitions of the treatment is not uncommon. Don't worry about it: just treat again until the muscle tests strong.

Sometimes it is not possible to clear the allergy and change the muscle response with at-home treatments. Any one of several factors may be interfering with the clearing process. These can be dealt with, but the process is more complex and requires the expertise of a trained BioSET™ practitioner. A referral list is posted on the BioSET™ Web site, at www. bioset-institute.com.

PART 2: THE NINETEEN POINTS

Using the same acupressure technique discussed above, stimulate the nineteen points shown in the illustrations on pages 178 and 179. These points are standard acupressure points designed to stimulate energy flow throughout the body. Have the subject continue to hold the vial(s) during this part of the procedure. This helps to clear any blockages in the electromagnetic energetic system of the body and assists in the treatment.

Begin Part 2 on the right side, with an acupressure point on the hand, and work your way through the points, following the list and diagrams that follow. Starting with the right side of the body, continue in a clockwise direction until you have made a complete circle. All the points have exactly the same location on both the right and left side and are paired, with the exception of one point, GV 20, on top of the head. The points are described below using acupressure designations from traditional Chinese medicine. End on the same point that you began with.

Description of the nineteen BioSET™ Acupressure Points

1. LI 4, right: Near the webbing between the thumb and index finger on the back of the hand.
2. LI 11, right: With the elbow bent, this point lies in the depression between the end of the elbow crease and the elbow.
3. TW 10, right: With the elbow bent, this point lies in the depression just above the elbow on the back of the arm.
4. BL 10, right: At the back of the head, about one inch on either side of the spine, in the center of the muscle just below the bony ridge at the base of the skull.
5. GV 20: To find this point, draw an imaginary line from the tip of one ear up and over the head to the tip of the other ear. The point is on the top of the head, exactly at the midpoint of this line.
6. BL 10, left: At the back of the head, about one inch on either side of the spine, in the center of the muscle just below the bony ridge at the base of the skull.
7. TW 10, left: With the elbow bent, this point lies in the depression just above the elbow on the back of the arm.
8. LI 11, left: With the elbow bent, this point lies in the depression between the end of the elbow crease and the elbow.
9. LI 4, left: Near the webbing between the thumb and index finger on the back of the hand.
10. BL 40, left: This point is in the middle of the large crease directly behind the knee.
11. ST 36, left: About two or three inches (about three or four fingers' width) directly below the lower edge of the kneecap, directly in line with the little toe.

12. SP6, left: On the inside of the leg, about two inches above the ankle-bone, in the soft tissue just behind the tibia (the larger of the two bones in the lower leg).

13. LIV 3, left: In the depression just between the first and second tarsal bones of the foot (big toe and second toe).

14. SP3, left: In the arch of the foot, closest to the big toe.

15. SP3, right: In the arch of the foot, closest to the big toe.

16. LIV 3, right: In the depression just between the first and second tarsal bones of the foot (big toe and second toe).

17. SP6, right: On the inside of the leg, about two inches above the ankle-bone, in the soft tissue just behind the tibia (the larger of the two bones in the lower leg).

18. ST 36, right: About two or three inches (about three or four fingers' width) directly below the lower edge of the kneecap, directly in line with the little toe.

19. BL 40, right: This point is in the middle of the large crease directly behind the knee.

Now have your subject rest comfortably for fifteen minutes with the sample still in her hand.

BIOSET™ SELF-TREATMENT

The procedure for performing treatments on yourself involves Part 2 only—acupressure on the nineteen points.

Stage 1. Testing. With the sample or vial in contact with your body, test yourself with the O-Ring method described on page 156. Use this method to identify possible food allergens for treatment.

Stage 2. The Nineteen Points. Since it is impossible for you to treat the back points yourself, simply skip Part 1 of the treatment; instead, repeat Part 2. Do the series six times. Repeat the series once every fifteen minutes over the course of approximately one and a half hours. Hold the samples

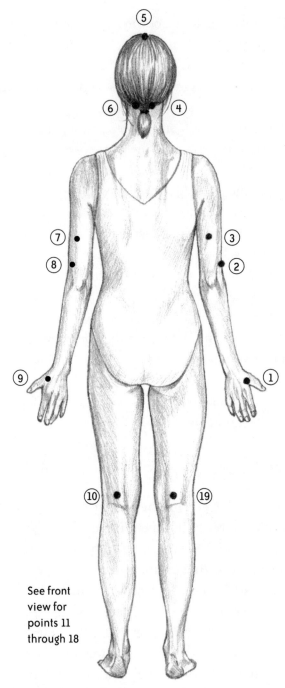

See front
view for
points 11
through 18

Acupressure points.

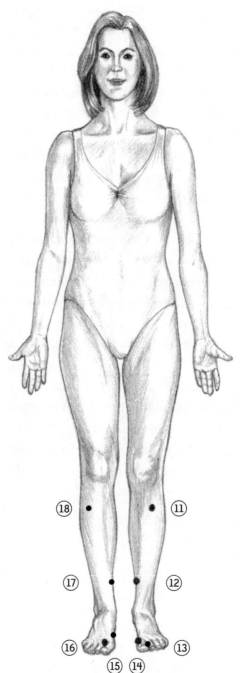

Acupressure points.

in your hand for the entire hour and a half. Since it can be impractical to try to hold the samples while engaging in a great deal of activity, do the self-treatments while engaging in sedentary activity such as watching TV or a movie, or reading.

Stage 3. Retest. At the end of the treatment cycle, retest yourself with the food allergen vial and the blood vial still in your hand, to make sure that you now test strong in response to the item.

Some foods may need to be treated more than once. Foods that have been bothersome for some time may need several complete treatments. Vicky, a former patient of mine and an avid self-treater, told me that it took her eleven BioSET™ self-treatments, one a day, to finally clear herself of a milk sensitivity. Now she is fully desensitized and able to eat all dairy products with no symptoms. If, after several treatments, you have not been successful, please consult a BioSET™ practitioner.

On occasion you may experience an allergic reaction to a food while eating it or immediately afterward. If it is not a severe reaction, you can use the BioSET™ allergy elimination technique on the spot to achieve a complete clearing, or at the very least to decrease your symptoms. For example, if you have just eaten a cookie and you are experiencing a headache, you can use another cookie to treat this reaction. Simply place a small piece of cookie in a glass and proceed with the BioSET™ treatment. This will usually reduce or completely eliminate the headache, and you probably will have little or no sensitivity to this cookie ever again.

9

Detoxification

We don't live and breathe in a clean, nourishing, and sustaining environment. Instead, we are assaulted daily by a toxic world in which there are fast-food restaurants on every corner, toxic food additives, canned goods, chemicals, prescription drugs, and radiation. Unfortunately, as Western civilization developed technologically, it sacrificed critical life supports, and now it seems that there is no escape. The soil is contaminated with pesticides and herbicides, and even our drinking water has become contaminated with toxic chemicals and microorganisms such as bacteria and parasites. Industrial wastes have exposed us to harmful substances such as hydrocarbons, phenols, and other chemicals.

Other common sources of toxins in everyday life include noise, stress and emotional trauma, poorly digested food, electromagnetic energy from high-voltage cables and household electronic devices such as computers and televisions, and environmental toxins such as heavy metals, pollens, industrial chemicals, pesticides, preservatives, smog, bacteria, parasites, and fungi.

Another source of toxins is the metabolic wastes that our own system cannot process and remove—for example, excess uric acid, free radicals (substances that can damage or kill cells), residues of medicinal and recreational drugs, and excess estrogen and cortisol.

When all these combinations of toxins assault the body, the immune system's capacity to protect our body's balance is overwhelmed. Food allergies are often the result. How do we discern the difference between toxicity and food allergies? Initially it is nearly impossible to do so. That is why the first step I take with my clients is a program of detoxification. Once the body has been detoxified, we can look at the symptoms that remain and match them to various food allergies.

HOW THE BODY NATURALLY DISPOSES OF TOXINS

Upon exposure to a toxin, the body attempts to eliminate the substance. Our bodies have many natural detoxification mechanisms. The organs that do most of this work are the skin, lungs, gastrointestinal tract, kidneys, and liver.

Biochemically, detoxification occurs in two phases. The first phase usually involves the transformation of toxic substances, such as chemicals, pesticides, or food additives. As a result of this process, however, additional toxic and reactive chemicals are created that need further detoxification. For example, the coal tar toxin in cigarette smoke is an inert substance until it is converted by enzymes into a harmful metabolite. This dangerous free radical can cause severe tissue damage, or even cancer, if not further transformed. During the second phase of detoxification, the body acts on these metabolites to further break them down, principally by increasing the body's ability to eliminate them through urine and bile. This process is of the utmost importance in preventing cellular damage and ill health.

When our organs of elimination are overtaxed, unable to keep up with this huge task, our body automatically calls upon our immune system for help. But sometimes even that is not enough. If our levels of toxic substances are too great, we become overloaded and our whole system becomes compromised. Our digestive system cannot function properly and our immune system is unable to efficiently fight those viruses and bacteria. This promotes premature aging, lack of sufficient energy, and poor enzyme production—all things that detract from the healthy functioning of each of our cells. We feel tired and depressed, and we have allergic reactions to foods that were no problem before.

When the body is in a state of homeostasis, it can accomplish detoxification efficiently. If you are struggling with food allergies, however, that could be an early warning sign that your system cannot adequately detoxify itself. In that case, intervention is needed. In fact, helping your body to detoxify is the first step toward freedom from food allergies.

HOW DO WE KNOW WHEN WE HAVE A TOXIC OVERLOAD?

Any substance that is harmful or dangerous to the body and distorts our natural homeostasis can be called a toxin. Therefore, if an individual is suffering from a toxic overload, she will manifest bodily imbalances. When the body's capacity to detoxify itself is exceeded, toxins are deposited both within and around the cells. This causes a wide variety of health problems that mimic many other, more serious diseases, such as rheumatoid arthritis and osteoarthritis, multiple sclerosis, depression, and autoimmune diseases. The symptoms of toxicity may take years to manifest after an initial exposure to a toxin, making it difficult to discern the real source of the symptoms and the actual problem.

I rarely see patients who do not have some kind of problem with toxins in their system. These substances are hard to avoid unless you are already aware of what causes toxicity and are actively doing some form of intervention or cleansing. Symptoms of toxicity that I commonly encounter in my own practice are headaches, muscle pain, fatigue, mental confusion, attention deficit hyperactivity disorder, rashes, exaggerated emotions, restlessness, irritability, nausea, swollen glands, joint aches, sudden hair loss, dizziness, and edema.

Detoxification is a primary and natural beginning to any healing process. One of the values of detoxification is that it gives a health care practitioner a clearer picture of what is actually happening in the body. This was certainly the case with Harry, a fifty-six-year-old man who came to see me recently. Harry had been seeking help from numerous doctors for many years. His symptoms included severe burning and itching over his entire body, irritability, insomnia, nagging headaches, and nausea. He would experience one or all of these symptoms daily.

Finally, one doctor suggested that Harry come to me. Harry had tried other allergy elimination programs over the years, but with no success. During his initial visit, Harry filled out an extensive questionnaire that led me to conclude that he was suffering from severe toxicity as well as allergies, and could benefit from a detoxification regimen. When I suggested this to him, he replied, "Dr. Cutler, no other physician has ever mentioned this possibility to me, and I am grateful." I first prescribed some homeopathic remedies that matched Harry's symptoms. When he returned two weeks later, all his symptoms had disappeared except for the headaches. I was then able to review his allergy tests to see if any food allergies might be the source of his headaches—which they were. After two months of BioSET™ allergy elimination treatments, Harry's headaches were a thing of the past. He was, in his own words, "as good as new."

☙ JARED'S STORY

Jared, a fourteen-year-old diagnosed with asthma, was brought to me by his parents, who had become completely frustrated with the general medical routine of asthma drugs. They felt that their son was getting worse, not better, and hoped that allergy treatments would be the answer.

Allergies are definitely a major cause of asthma, and my results treating asthma sufferers of all age groups have been extraordinary. After I had spent some time reviewing Jared's diet, however, I learned that he lived on fast-food lunches, such as hot dogs, sausages, and hamburgers, which include food additives, food coloring, and preservatives, and soft drinks with high sugar content. His diet lacked wholesome, organic, balanced meals. I concluded that he needed some nutritional education and a period of detoxifying and cleansing. After having Jared fill out a detoxification questionnaire and reviewing the results, I recommended that he take a homeopathic remedy for gentle cleansing. I also discussed some dietary recommendations with him, including skipping the soft drinks and, at least three days a week, packing a school lunch that included a whole-grain sandwich made with something like organic turkey, some vegetable sticks, and springwater.

Jarel agreed to these changes, and when he returned in three weeks, he looked completely different. His asthma had disappeared and his acne had improved. He said he felt more energetic than he had in years, and he needed less sleep to feel rested. I then began giving him BioSET™ allergy elimination treatments. Now, three years later, he does not require any type of medication.

DETOXIFYING BY MAKING LIFESTYLE CHANGES

Fully healing from food allergies means learning about the process of detoxification and making certain important changes in your lifestyle. Even small changes can go a long way toward helping to cleanse your system. In this section are several suggestions about things you can do at home to detoxify yourself and substances and situations you should avoid. At the end of this chapter I have also included a detoxification appraisal questionnaire to help you to evaluate your level of toxicity.

FASTING AND JUICING

There are many different methods of detoxification that we can make a part of our daily lives. Our bodies function twenty-four hours each day, and in the long run, eight hours of sleep per night is often not really enough for them to adequately rest and regenerate. For this reason, it is important that we provide our bodies with additional opportunities for rest and cleansing, preferably several times a year.

One activity that we can do regularly is fasting. Fasting helps the body to heal and to resist diseases, infections, and toxins. It frees up the energy of the colon so that this energy can be used in other places. Most important, fasting gives the body an opportunity to return to its natural state of homeostasis. During a fast, the body produces new, healthy cells to replace old, depleted ones.

Many people adopt a schedule of consuming only liquids one day each week, or for a three-day period once a month. Some even fast for as long as three to ten days at a time on just vegetable broth and vegetable juices.

In order to get the most out of your fruit and vegetable drinks, it is best to juice the produce yourself rather than buying the juice commercially. In order to ensure that your juices are pure and full of nutrients, you should use as much organically grown produce as possible. This keeps harmful pesticides and chemical residues from ending up in your juice. If you are unable to obtain organically grown fruits and vegetables, make sure you peel or thoroughly wash your produce, using a vegetable brush to remove chemical residues and waxes. Most health food stores carry vegetable washes that help remove any residues.

The juices I have used most often over the years are beet, carrot, cabbage, celery, cucumber, kale, parsley, turnip, spinach, and watercress. I do not recommend using carrot juice on its own, as carrots are higher in natural sugars than other vegetables, and since most individuals are sensitive to sugar, carrot juice can compromise inner balance and effective detoxification. However, when used in moderation, it is excellent for sweetening other juices. Strongly flavored vegetables, such as broccoli, celery, onions, parsley, rutabagas, and turnips, should be used in small amounts.

Green drinks, which use a lot of leafy green vegetables, raw sprouts, and grasses as their primary ingredients, also cleanse the body of pollutants and have a rejuvenating effect. The chlorophyll in these drinks helps to purify the blood and detoxify the body. Green juices can be made using alfalfa sprouts, celery, dandelion greens, spinach, cabbage, and wheatgrass. I sometimes sweeten my green drink using carrot juice and apple juice. Green juices have great health benefits, but they are very potent and should be consumed only in moderation. This means no more than eight to ten ounces a day.

An excellent green drink recipe is:

1 beet, including top
1 large handful of spinach
1 large handful of kale
4–5 carrots

Put all ingredients through a juicer.

During fasting, you should drink at least eight glasses of liquid each day. It is also wise to use distilled water to dilute juices from fresh fruits and vegetables, to prevent your digestive system from being overloaded. It is good to take vitamin and mineral supplements when eating normally, but do not take them while fasting because they can interfere with the cleansing process.

If you prefer a hot drink during fasting, I recommend making vegetable broths. Here is the recipe for my favorite vegetable broth:

3 stalks celery
2 large red potatoes, unpeeled
3 medium beets with tops
4 carrots
1 onion
1 clove of garlic

Put the vegetables in a pot and add water to cover. Simmer, covered, for 45 minutes. Remove the vegetables, blend the broth and any remaining vegetables in a blender, and drink it when it has cooled down.

Once you are ready to end your fast, you should return to solid foods gradually, over a period of three to four days. Start out by eating lightly, and always chew your foods well. This enhances the digestive process.

Do not undertake a fast longer than three days without medical supervision.

CHANGING THE WAY YOU EAT

Changing one's diet is another great way to detoxify the body and return it to balance. One good example of an eating plan that helps the body to detoxify is a macrobiotic diet. This type of diet emphasizes eating only those foods grown in the area in which you live. For example, if you live in the northern United States or Canada, you should avoid eating tropical fruits. A macrobiotic diet also includes as many whole foods as possible, such as brown rice, millet, whole rye, and other foods that have not been subjected to significant processing. Ideally, these foods should be cooked in such a way as to preserve their nutrients. Optimal cooking involves steaming foods, rather than boiling or baking them, and poaching instead of frying.

The classic macrobiotic diet consists of 50–60 percent whole grains, 20–30 percent locally grown vegetables, 5–10 percent beans and sea vegetables, 5–10 percent soups, and 5 percent condiments and other foods. You should avoid highly processed foods, sugar, dairy products, red meat, poultry, fish, and commercial salt. Use sea salt instead, because it contains more minerals.

Here are some recipes that I enjoy and recommend to my patients:

MISO SOUP

Makes 4 servings

> 2 dried shiitake mushrooms
> 4 c filtered water
> 1/3 block firm tofu, cubed
> 3 tbsp miso (organic barley or traditional barley, or red)
> 1 tsp organic toasted sesame oil
> Green onions, sliced for garnish

Soak shiitakes in 1 cup of the filtered water for 20 minutes. Remove and slice thinly. Combine soaking water and remaining 3 cups of filtered water, bring to a boil, and add the shiitakes. Reduce heat and simmer for 5 minutes. Add the tofu to the stock and heat through. Make a thin paste of miso with a small amount of stock, add it to the pot, and cook on low heat for 2 minutes. Add sesame oil, garnish with green onions, and serve.

MASHED POTATOES WITH MISO GRAVY

Makes 4 servings

> 3 medium boiling potatoes, cut up
> ³/₄ c filtered water
> ¹/₂ c soy milk
> Sea salt and black pepper, to taste
> 1 tsp olive oil
> 1 onion, minced
> 1 clove garlic, minced
> 2 tsp miso (organic barley, brown rice, or red)

Boil potatoes in salted water until tender, then drain. Put them through a rice or food mill or mash them with a fork. Add milk, salt and pepper, and set aside. Heat the oil in the skillet and sauté the onion over medium heat until lightly browned. Add garlic and sauté about 30 more seconds. Add the miso mix and stir until thickened. Pour over mashed potatoes and serve immediately.

TOFU SALAD

Makes 2–4 servings

> 1 block firm tofu
> 3 tbsp miso (barley, white, or chickpea)
> 1–2 tbsp pickled ginger
> 1 tsp juice from pickled ginger
> 2 tsp tahini
> 1 tsp organic toasted sesame oil
> 1 stalk celery, diced small
> 2 scallions, thinly sliced
> 1 c chopped sprouts (preferably daikon sprouts)

Press tofu under a weighted plate for 30 minutes to release excess moisture. Blot with towels. Combine the miso with the pickled ginger, a teaspoon of ginger juice, the tahini, and the sesame oil. Crumble the tofu with your hands into a large bowl. Add the miso mixture and combine thoroughly. Stir in the celery, scallions, and sprouts. Spread on toasted whole-grain bread or stuff into a tortilla with lettuce and carrots.

ADZUKI BEAN AND WINTER SQUASH STEW

Makes 6–8 servings

> $1^{1}/_{2}$ c dry adzuki beans
> 6 c filtered water
> 3 c winter squash, cubed
> 2 tsp miso (organic barley, red, or brown rice)
> 1-in piece of fresh ginger
> 1 tsp organic toasted sesame oil

Soak the beans overnight. Discard the soaking water and bring the beans to a boil in 6 cups of filtered water. Lower the heat and cook in a pressure cooker for 20 minutes, or 60 minutes on the stovetop. When the beans are almost tender, add the winter squash and simmer for 20 minutes or until the squash is tender. Using some of the bean liquid, dilute the miso and add it to the pot. Peel and grate the ginger, then, using your hands, squeeze out the juice. Add the juice and the sesame oil to the pot and heat for 5 minutes, stirring occasionally.

DAIRY-FREE PESTO

Makes approx. 3/4 c pesto

> 1 c tightly packed fresh basil, leaves only
> 2–4 cloves garlic, peeled
> $^{1}/_{4}$ c fresh parsley, destemmed
> $^{1}/_{4}$ c walnuts or pine nuts, toasted
> 2–4 tbsp miso (organic barley, white, or chickpea)
> $^{1}/_{4}$–$^{1}/_{2}$ c extra-virgin olive oil

Combine the first 5 ingredients in a blender or food processor. Very slowly trickle the olive oil through top of the machine with the motor running until the desired consistency is reached. This may be smooth or chunky, according to your liking. Serve with vegetables, or stir a spoonful into soup for a flavorful treat.

MISO HUMMUS

Makes 2–4 servings

> *1 c chickpeas, cooked*
> *2 cloves garlic*
> *2 tbsp tahini*
> *1 lemon, juiced (1¹/₂ tbsp juice)*

Blend all the ingredients in a food processor or blender. Serve as a dip for pita bread, crackers, or veggies, or as a delicious sandwich spread with red onion, lettuce, and tomato.

These are just a few of my favorite recipes. You can find many more in *American Macrobiotic Cuisine,* by Meredith McCarthy, and *Aveline Kushi's Complete Guide to Macrobiotic Cooking,* by Aveline Kushi.

FOODS TO AVOID

If you want to have a healthy, toxin-free body, there are certain foods that it is important to avoid, such as:

- Refined sugars and refined carbohydrates
- Caffeine, an addictive substance that inhibits the body's natural ability to detoxify
- Alcohol, another addictive substance and one that causes degeneration of our cells
- A high salt intake, which can cause a deficiency of potassium, an important mineral for healthy muscles, including the muscles of the heart
- Artificial sweeteners, food additives, and food coloring
- Foods that have been sprayed with pesticides and fungicides, which are carcinogenic and toxic

It is also important to avoid eating any genetically altered foods. These are called genetically modified organisms, or GMOs, and are sold in supermarkets across the country. In recent years, many grains and produce have been altered to incorporate different characteristics or to improve shelf life. For example, in the 1990s, the U.S. Department of Agriculture gave the okay to Calgene, Inc., to produce a tomato that takes longer than usual to rot. It seems that the Campbell Soup Company financed this development and was going to market the new tomato, but decided against it because they felt their brand stood for wholesome ingredients, and GMOs are not considered wholesome and natural. Gerber baby foods has also stopped using GMOs.

So if you see signs in supermarkets that say "genetically modified organisms," you will know that the attractive label actually means "This food is unsafe to eat!"

EXERCISE

A systematic program of exercise is essential to detoxification because it strengthens the cardiovascular system. Lack of exercise causes toxins to build up in our bodies. Studies have shown that exercise can actually speed up the removal of toxins and waste materials and increase the flow of nutrient-carrying blood to every cell. Exercise can also help lower blood pressure and prevent heart attacks. A consistent program of exercise restores lung power and improves bone structure and muscle flexibility. It can also aid in weight reduction and shorten the duration of allergic reactions.

Exercise has many emotional and psychological benefits as well. It has been shown to improve mental health, decrease anger and hostility, reduce stress, elevate mood because of the release of endorphins (substances secreted by the brain to help mask pain and bring about a feeling of euphoria) it triggers, and improve memory and learning potential.

Aerobic exercise, such as brisk walking, jogging, or swimming, is one of the best forms of exercise. It should be done for a minimum of thirty to forty-five minutes at least three times a week. I have found moderate aerobic exercise done consistently over a longer period of time to be more effective than strenuous exercise done in short bursts.

Brisk walking is the very best aerobic exercise because the heart works at a safe rate, which promotes cardiovascular fitness. A regular walking program can enhance endurance, increase oxygen uptake, improve circulation and muscle tone, promote weight loss, and release toxins through perspiration. Walking has been known to help with emotional cleansing, reducing anxiety, stress, and depression.

If you choose to take up brisk walking and you are pollen-sensitive, find an area that does not have heavy vegetation. In many places, a high concentration of pollen is a seasonal phenomenon, so you can pick and choose your times and areas. Chemically sensitive individuals should find an area away from traffic.

Running is another popular method of exercise. It is estimated that there are over thirty-three million runners in America. Running has always been my favorite form of exercise as it improves lung capacity, strengthens the muscles and bones, reduces body fat, and improves circulation. I feel an instant positive mood change when I run. But running is not something that I, as a chiropractor, recommend to most of my patients. Because it is a high-impact exercise, running can be a risk for those with a history of knee, hip, and ankle problems or a lower back condition.

If you do choose to run, know that warming up by stretching beforehand is critical to prevent sprains, strains, and tendinitis. Burning pain in your muscles while exercising and extended cramping afterward are clear indications that your method of exercise is too strenuous.

Regular long-distance swimming produces the same benefits as running, cycling, or cross-country skiing. One advantage of swimming is that you become fit very rapidly. You can get into top shape by swimming just twice a week for fifteen minutes. Exercise in the pool may take the form of swimming laps; running, walking, or jumping in the water; or using a kickboard. The water acts as a giant cushion for these activities, absorbing the shock of the movements and providing low-impact exercise. Because water has more resistance than air, walking or running in water makes your leg muscles, heart, and lungs work hard even though your speed for these activities will be slower. Water exercise sessions are available at some public pools.

Pool water can be a threat to asthmatics and those who are sensitive to chlorine. Wear goggles to help protect your eyes. A nose clip will prevent water from entering the nose, and showering immediately after the swimming sessions is also useful.

Cycling is another popular aerobic exercise. It is not a weight-bearing activity and therefore is less stressful to your joints. Bicycling can be as beneficial as running, increasing circulation and the flow of oxygen to your cells and helping to eliminate toxins. Stationary bicycles offer more environmental control and safety than outdoor bicycles. The best stationary bicycles are those that exercise your arms as well as your legs.

There are other exercise systems that are as effective as aerobic exercise for cleansing and detoxifying. Two of the most popular are the martial arts disciplines chi kung and tai chi. Chi kung, also known as qigong, is a Chinese term applied to the many different forms of exercise that work with the chi (breath). *Kung* means "discipline" or "one who spends time practicing." Therefore, *chi kung* can be interpreted to mean "the practice of proper breathing." With practice, you can feel the chi energy flowing through the body. These exercises cause a flushing of the body's toxins and waste materials.

Chi kung exercises also provide active motions to enhance and strengthen the body as a whole. The Chinese use chi kung for treating chronic diseases.

Tai chi is another form of Chinese exercise. Tai chi is a series of continuous, slow, fluid, and graceful movements that are performed in a relaxed manner, with the knees slightly bent and the body in a straight and upright posture. Described as "meditation in motion," tai chi involves a series of harmonious movements during which one focuses on the breath. When correctly performed, tai chi can stimulate circulation, detoxify, relax the joints, and encourage mental relaxation. People who practice tai chi often become profoundly dedicated to this form of exercise because of its resulting feelings of well-being.

Yoga, an ancient system of breathing movements and postures, has become very popular over the last couple of decades. Yoga not only brings tranquillity of body and mind, freeing us from unwanted stress, it also enhances the flexibility of the spine, releases muscular tension, and increases the circulation to our organs and glands. Many different forms of yoga have been developed over the centuries in response to climate, culture, body constitution, lifestyle, and the physical environment. Each form has its own particular emphasis but also incorporates facets of the other forms. One of the more physical forms of yoga is hatha yoga, which concentrates on postures and movements that encourage the body to stretch and tone. Kundalini yoga concentrates on the spinal column, strengthening and balancing the nervous system. Pranayama yoga focuses on breathing and the strengthening and balancing of the respiratory system.

I am in favor of all forms of yoga. Not only can yoga realign or even prevent spinal misalignments, it reverses the effects of gravity's downward pull on the vital organs and glands in the body. Inversion exercises, such as the shoulder stand, increase the blood supply to organs and glands. Other postures stimulate the kidneys, liver, stomach, colon, and pancreas to promote cleansing and purification.

Since there are many other types of yoga classes, I suggest choosing the yoga that feels best for you. Ask around, visit a class, and talk with the instructors. If you are seeking to learn yoga as a tool to rid your body of toxins, even a home video will be effective.

MASSAGE

Massage is another excellent adjunct to detoxification. Our bodies respond both externally and internally to friction on the skin, pressure on deeper tissues, and sensory input around the joints. Most physicians believe that our bodies rely on the movement of fluids to function well, and massage is an effective means of promoting fluid circulation. To survive and function, every cell must continuously receive nutrients, water, and oxygen while toxic wastes are being taken away. This cycle of receiving and expelling involves circulation.

Massage improves circulation. Lazy muscles are encouraged to work, and connective tissue is softened and stretched. Massage also facilitates cleansing and the removal of waste materials from the body. It improves blood and lymph circulation, increases the oxygen supply to cells, and eliminates excess fluid in the muscles and tissues.

Any type of massage directly affects the nerves, organs, and circulation and indirectly affects the body as a whole. Massage can help the body and mind to cope with stress and pain. We all know how a soothing, comforting touch affects both children and adults, alleviating shock, distress, or fear. The pathways carrying sensations of touch to the brain are thicker, faster, and more numerous than the pathways that carry pain. When the body is distracted from pain by touch, it is able to relax tense muscles. And when pain is lessened, a person is able to better evaluate a stressful situation.

All massage techniques work by stimulating specific receptors in the skin, resulting in a particular reaction, depending upon the type of massage used. Let me caution you that some physical conditions preclude vigorous, stimulating, and/or deep massage. If you are under a physician's care, always request an evaluation before getting a massage.

The basic types of massage are soft-tissue massage, lymphatic massage, fascia and connective tissue massage, massage of the meridians, and energy and healing touch work.

Swedish massage is the most familiar style of soft-tissue bodywork. It involves treatment of the entire external body except for the reproductive organs and body orifices. A person receiving this type of massage is always draped and may undress to the degree that is personally comfortable. Oil, powder, or alcohol are the mediums most often used to help the therapist's hands glide smoothly over the skin surface. Swedish massage stretches the limbs and actively stimulates the skin and soft tissue.

Manual lymphatic massage should be practiced only by a trained professional. In this large-surface type of massage the skin is kneaded, never stroked. Because the effect of lymphatic massage is largely mechanical, displacing fluids and the substances they carry, the techniques must be executed precisely. The more exact the technique, the more effective the results.

In *fascia massage*, the fascia—the part of our bodies that fastens the muscles to the bones and the bones to the joints, surrounds every nerve and vessel, holds all internal structures in place, and envelops the body as a whole—is massaged with direct pressure through squeezing, stretching, and contorting. This type of massage moves large amounts of toxins and wastes out of the intercellular fluids and into the bloodstream, where they can be eliminated.

Rolfing, another method of deep massage, uses fingers, knuckles, forearms, elbows, and sometimes even special tools to stretch or exert pressure on the body's connective tissues in an effort to energize and reshape them. This pressure and stretching, carefully applied at specific points and in specific directions, softens and lengthens the connective tissues to make them more malleable. This promotes detoxification and cleansing of the system. Rolfing also addresses the structural properties of the connective tissue.

Shiatsu massage, a form of acupressure developed in Japan, has been described as a dance over and along the meridians of the body. The practitioner uses her body weight rather than her muscle strength to allow her hands or fingers to penetrate into the meridians. Pressure is applied rhythmically and in a perpendicular direction. The practitioner uses the balls of the fingers, the thumbs, and the base of the thumbs in a combination of eleven specific positions.

Shiatsu massage can help to reduce muscle tension by stimulating points along the meridians that are related to particular muscles or joints.

This technique is effective for overall cleansing of the body as well as specific ailments such as migraines, stiff neck, and sciatica.

Reflexology is a Chinese method of foot massage. It is referred to as a "zone therapy" because the specific pressure points stimulated on the feet reflect the entire body. Each foot represents one-half of the body. Treatment consists of using the thumbs to apply firm pressure. Working on these reflexes can cleanse the body, relieve headaches, clear congested sinuses, reduce the pain of menstrual cramps, ease backaches, and reduce swelling.

DRINKING ENOUGH WATER

Adequate water intake is necessary for effective cleansing. I recommend taking a large sip of water every thirty minutes and drinking a whole glass twenty to thirty minutes before eating your meal in order to obtain the appropriate daily water intake. Bottled water is recommended.

If you prefer not to drink bottled water, then you should consider a water filter to remove unwanted contaminants from tap water. Although there are many types of filters on the market, most of them do not remove all undesirable elements from our drinking water. For that reason I refer you to Appendix 1 for more information on water filtration systems.

I recommend using safe water not only for drinking but for cooking, brushing your teeth, washing fresh food, and bathing and hand washing.

BREATHING

Breathing, one of the only functions of the body that we can perform both consciously and unconsciously, is an important and very basic cleansing method. It can help cleanse the body both physically and mentally. Breathing is also directly connected to our emotional states, all of which affect the speed, depth, and regularity with which we breathe. For example, anger, which makes us take quick, shallow breaths, can be calmed by breathing slowly, deeply, quietly, and regularly. Most people do not realize that stressful emotions can limit the body's ability to detoxify. For this reason, learning some appropriate breathing techniques can be profoundly cleansing.

One detoxifying breathing technique, described in *Radical Healing* by Rudolph Ballentine, M.D., is called diaphragmatic breathing. To do this exercise, lie on your stomach on a firm surface such as the floor with your forehead resting comfortably on your crossed arms, or lie on your back with a three-pound object, such as a large snap-seal bag filled with sand, on your belly. The goal of this exercise is to practice effortless breathing in the midriff region rather than in the belly or the chest. This is achieved by simply holding in your abdominal muscles as you inhale so that the lower edges of your rib cage are pushed outward, expanding the diaphragm. This breathing exercise promotes calmness and quietness and releases blocked energy pathways, promoting cleansing and revitalization. It also targets emotional cleansing, helping to release tension.

The more air we breathe in and out of our lungs, the healthier we are. The delivery of oxygen and removal of carbon dioxide determines the efficiency of functioning for all body systems. The body cannot cleanse itself, heal itself, or maintain life without the oxygen supplied by breathing. The motions of respiration mechanically pump lymphatic fluid and assist circulation. If breathing is restricted, fluid collects, causing edema and the buildup of waste products from cellular metabolism. If as we go through our stressful, chaotic, activity-filled days, we could all just remember to periodically take in a deep breath and release it slowly, we would derive great detoxifying benefits from breathing.

DRY SKIN BRUSHING

Dry skin brushing is an effective tool for skin cleansing and detoxification. This technique involves briskly brushing the entire body with a dry vegetable-fiber or other soft-bristle brush before showering or bathing. Begin with the soles of your feet and work up to the top of your legs in large broad strokes. When you get to the top part of your body, brush from the palms of the hands toward the shoulders. Always aim toward the lymph nodes, located in the groin and underarm areas. Never brush the nipples or the face, and always brush toward the heart when doing the chest and back area. I recommend brushing for about five minutes three times a week. This greatly improves skin cleansing beyond the benefits of just a bath or shower alone.

DETOXIFYING BATHS AND SAUNAS

Detoxification baths help eliminate toxins by activating fluid movement in the tissues and increasing perspiration. I have always favored Epsom salts baths because they promote relaxation and calmness. These salts work as a counterirritant on the skin to increase blood supply. The sulfur content of Epsom salts also aids in detoxification. You should begin with ¼ cup of Epsom salts in the bath and gradually increase the amount with each bath until you are using 4 cups per tub of water.

Herbal and clay baths. Although clay is most frequently used in compresses or packs, the drawing action of clay in the bath also aids in detoxification. Use ½ cup of betonite clay to a tub of water (soaking flat container overnight to dissolve). There are several types of clay on the market and all are appropriate for bathing. This betonite clay is sold specifically for bathing and will not clog up your drain, but use sparingly to prevent this from occurring.

Saunas have also been used therapeutically for detoxification. A sauna is a relatively airtight room with wooden platforms and benches. The air is kept fresh by a special ventilation system that preheats outside air before it enters the sauna. There are two basic types of saunas, dry or moist, and both have a temperature of about 140–150 degrees Fahrenheit. A sauna is a very effective tool for releasing stored toxins from the cells.

When looking for a sauna to use in your detoxification program, I suggest finding a dry sauna that has been constructed to be environmentally safe, with air cleaners attached to the air circulation units. Although most commercial saunas found in health clubs are safe, some tend to be too hot and/or have inadequate levels of oxygen. For this reason, it always helps to ask the club management about their sauna. I recommend dry saunas because they increase sweating and speed detoxification. While sweating in the sauna, be sure to replace the fluids you are losing—drink plenty of water, both while you are in the sauna and afterward, to keep your kidneys flushing out the toxins. After completing a sauna, allow yourself a period of rest. The body needs a quiet time to adjust and rebalance itself.

CLEANSING THE ORGANS OF ELIMINATION

Our primary detoxification organs are the liver and the colon. During times of stress and acute overload, cleansing these organs will help to restore their optimal function.

The liver is a major factor in the elimination of toxic wastes. It processes all the chemicals we are exposed to daily, such as pollution, drugs, or cleaning products. The liver also metabolizes hormones, such as estrogen, that are used in regulating the body's processes. If the liver is unable to process estrogen adequately due to a toxic overload, excess estrogen is the result. This can lead to high blood pressure and breast, uterine, or vaginal cancer. The liver also metabolizes testosterone. Overly high levels of this hormone can cause aggressiveness and mood swings as well as excessive sexual energy. Because the liver also filters the blood, an overburdened liver will not be able to adequately eliminate toxins from the blood. These unfiltered toxins can then infiltrate the liver cells, causing irreversible damage.

A poorly functioning liver can cause poor digestion, gas, constipation, soreness in the liver area, skin problems such as acne or psoriasis, emotional excesses, and unmetabolized toxins throughout the body, which can lead to disease. If you have several of these symptoms, you might consider a liver cleanse to help stimulate the elimination of toxic wastes from the body. I use a liver enzyme made from an herbal enzyme formula

(WellZyme Liver Cleanse; see Appendix 1) that helps to increase liver detoxification as well as restoration of its function. Other factors that can stimulate liver detoxification are minimizing protein intake; using only small amounts of unsaturated fats; eating foods such as garlic, onions, and broccoli; reducing intake of refined sugar; and moderately eating bitter green vegetables such as endive, collard, dock, and dandelion.

One of the best liver cleansers that I have found is a coffee enema. Coffee enemas are useful in ridding the body of toxins and accumulated waste products. A coffee enema is a low-volume enema that mainly stays in the end of the colon, the area where the colon and the liver are connected through the circulatory system. Toxins in this part of the colon are sent to the liver for detoxification rather than being circulated throughout the body. The shorter the amount of time that waste spends in this portion of the bowel, the smaller the amount of toxins that will wind up in the liver. A coffee enema can speed up the emptying of the bowel, increasing liver detoxification. Individuals who are very sensitive to caffeine are usually not affected because the caffeine goes only into the colon-liver circulation area, not into the entire system. Warning: People who have gallstones should not take enemas.

A healthy colon is also of the utmost importance in detoxification. A colon that is toxic or not performing optimally causes backup and fermentation of fecal material. When this happens, bacterial overgrowth develops, making the system toxic. This overgrowth can cause many symptoms, from migraines to sciatica to psychological disorders. Eventually the very integrity of our cells will be affected, limiting their ability to produce energy and fight disease.

Ultimately, good digestion is the key to good colon health. I strongly believe that if you take measures to chew and digest your food sufficiently, take supplemental enzymes and probiotics, eat a balanced diet that is suited to your individual needs, and drink enough water, your colon will remain healthy.

HOMEOPATHY AS A TREATMENT FOR DETOXIFICATION

Used by themselves or along with the detoxification methods described above, homeopathic remedies can help you to achieve detoxification quickly and effectively. I often use them in my own practice.

Homeopathy is a medical system developed two hundred years ago by Dr. Samuel Hahnemann, a German physician. The system is based on the philosophy "Let like be cured with like." Dr. Hahnemann felt that the body's responses to illness are an effort to heal itself, so giving a person a remedy that caused those same symptoms might actually help to boost the healing process. Hahnemann developed a system of homeopathic remedies based on this idea. He also believed that what is really being treated is a person's "vital force," the body's overall energy and vitality. The change in vital force determines the success of the homeopathic remedy given to the patient. When Hahnemann experimented with different potencies of his remedies, he found that the more-diluted substances had fewer side effects and acted longer and more deeply on the body, and thus were more effective.

As I have worked with eliminating the food allergies of thousands of patients over the years, I have gotten the best and longest-lasting results when my clients take a homeopathic remedy to assist them in cleansing the body. These remedies are most efficient in the beginning stages of healing. They work quickly and deeply, cause very few side effects, and are not highly allergenic. While they gently and effectively cleanse the system, they also treat the body's vital force and energy. Once someone takes a homeopathic remedy, he can feel symptoms decreasing almost immediately.

Homeopathic detoxification preparations stimulate the cells to release toxic residue. Once this process occurs, the body will begin to filter out this residue through the liver and colon. Sometimes, depending upon the toxic load, a person can experience adverse reactions, such as an increased need for sleep, anxiety, nervousness, bad breath, frequent urination, or softer stool. After the elimination process is complete, most people feel an increase in energy, a heightened feeling of well-being, and a greater resistance to colds and flu. (Additional information on homeopathic detoxification is provided in Appendix 1.)

One of my clients, Joselyn, a twenty-eight-year-old teacher, was so plagued by chronic fatigue that she was barely able to teach her eight-year-old students. Shortly after starting treatment with me, she faxed a letter to my office. It said, "Dear Dr. Cutler, I've been on your homeopathic remedy for nine days now, and I have more energy today than I've had in two years. I am encouraged."

THE SECRETS OF DETOXIFICATION IN DAILY LIFE

This chapter would not be complete without sharing some important factors for the prevention of toxicity.

Meg, a client, walked into my office recently, looked me in the eye, and said, "Dr. Cutler, I feel so good and I have so much energy. How can I remain this healthy and energetic?"

I thought for a while and then said, "Meg, what has been the most important information you have gained over this past month?"

Without hesitation, she said, "I haven't eaten any cheese or sugar, and I don't crave it. If it hadn't been for the homeopathics, digestive enzymes, and allergy treatments, I would not have been able to do this. But what else can I do to continue to feel this way?"

So I spent some time with Meg and told her what I am about to tell you—some secrets to help prevent toxicity.

DETOXIFYING FROM TRAUMA AND STRESS

A great deal has been written about trauma, stress, and the suppression of emotions as a source of toxicity and cause of disease. Since emotional stress has a significant impact upon the health of our bodies, it is important to acknowledge and address it.

Our conscious mind might have suppressed and forgotten our psychological traumas, but our subconscious and our cells remember. These traumatic memories wear down the body and our immune, endocrine, and nervous systems. The BioSET™ allergy elimination technique provides a means for the clearing of these emotional wounds. This, however, is not the kind of treatment that can be done at home. Rather, it needs to be taken care of by a skilled BioSET™ practitioner.

To avoid the buildup of toxicity through emotional distress, taking preventative measures is crucial. For example, counseling and psychotherapy are helpful as tools for the cleansing and destressing of both our minds and our bodies. I have also used homeopathic flower remedies for emotional trauma, abuse, and stress. Keeping a journal either daily or during times of stress is another great tool to promote emotional health. Record happy experiences as well as problematic and disturbing ones.

Laughter is another powerful tool for cleansing and clearing. Norman Cousins, the author of *Anatomy of an Illness*, discusses how laughter and love are very therapeutic. We can make ourselves laugh by watching a funny movie, listening to humorous tapes, reading funny books, or even spending some time with a young child who makes us smile and laugh.

ELIMINATING ELECTROMAGNETIC STRESS IN YOUR HOME

Electromagnetic fields can be another cause of stress. To minimize the effects of electromagnetic stress and toxicity in your home, there are some simple precautions that are important to follow. First of all, purchase a home that is a long distance from transformers and high-voltage wires. Second, keep your exposure to electrical appliances as limited as possible. Locate your bedroom as far away as you can from the area where electric current enters into your house. Keep a minimal number of electric appliances in your bedroom, and do not sleep with any of them plugged in. Do not use electric blankets, heating pads, or the heater in water beds. Use a shield over your computer screen. If you have fluorescent light fixtures, use full-spectrum lightbulbs.

AVOIDING TOXICITY IN THE WORKPLACE

All of us are regularly exposed to toxins and other chemicals in our workplaces. A simple solution is to make sure that there is adequate ventilation. Properly placed exhaust fans, chemical hoods, and adequate air exchange will all increase safety in the work area. Air cleaners may be a necessity in heavily polluted areas. Information on air filters is listed in Appendix 1. Even with adequate ventilation, it may still be necessary to install activated-charcoal filters to remove chemicals from the air. Wearing charcoal masks or respirators can protect workers exposed to chemicals.

MAKING SURE OUR CHILDREN'S SCHOOLS ARE NOT TOXIC ENVIRONMENTS

Children are a joy to be around, and it is our responsibility to keep them healthy and happy. Unfortunately, our children can be exposed to many serious toxins in their school environment. As parents, we must increase our awareness of the quality of their school environment, especially if they are attending a new school in a new area. Is the school near power lines? Are the children being exposed to excessive mold, dust, or toxic chemicals?

The following measures are useful to help protect our children:

- The air in new school buildings can contain formaldehyde, which is off-gassed from new building materials, so supply your child's classroom with plants, such as Boston ferns and palms, and buy an air cleaner. I bought an air cleaner for my child's classroom last year to reduce the mold that was obvious on the curtains. All the children coughed less that year.
- If possible, transfer your child to another school if there are high-voltage power lines nearby.
- The use of lead in both new plumbing and plumbing repairs is illegal at present, so old parts containing lead should be replaced.
- Request that your school use full-spectrum lights.
- Inquire about the pesticide-spraying schedule for plants surround-

ing the school, and keep your child home the day the pesticide is being applied.

Although keeping ourselves, our families, and our environment as toxin-free as possible requires an investment of time and perhaps even money, it is well worth the effort. Detoxification is a critical factor in health care. If you use this chapter to guide you in your understanding of toxicity and detoxification, I guarantee that you will reap many benefits.

10

Enzyme Therapy

As I was leaving my clinic one afternoon, I was again reminded of the healing benefits of supplementing our diet with plant enzymes.

Jack, a forty-six-year-old man, had recently visited my clinic complaining of symptoms of severe fatigue and sinus congestion. During our initial conversation, which lasted an hour and fifteen minutes, he said more than once that he did not remember a time when he had been able to breathe through his nose. He could not smell or taste well, and he occasionally suffered from painful headaches.

I have met many people, young and old, who suffer from sinus congestion, and I have found that this problem very often stems from poor digestion and food allergies. As I do with each new patient, I began by evaluating Jack's digestive stress, having him fill out an in-depth questionnaire (similar to the self-diagnostic one that appears at the end of this chapter). I then performed an enzyme evaluation. After these testing procedures were completed, I discovered that Jack was not digesting fats and proteins very well. I prescribed a supplemental plant enzyme that would help with the predigestion of these foods and a probiotic enzyme formula that contained lactobacilli to aid in reestablishing a healthy environment in his gut.

A week later, when Jack came in for his first allergy elimination treatment, he was filled with enthusiasm and looked like a new man. He said, "Dr. Cutler, I want to shake your hand. I began taking those enzymes the very next morning and have never missed a dose. Since then, I've had more energy than I can remember. And I've had moments when I could actually taste and smell well. For the first time in years, I could smell my morning pot of coffee brewing."

HOW OUR BODIES ARE NOURISHED

Before we can understand the importance of the role enzymes can play in our health, we first need to take a look at what our bodies take in to nourish themselves.

THE NUTRIENTS: FATS, PROTEIN, AND CARBOHYDRATES

Good nutritional management requires that we control our consumption of fats, protein, and carbohydrates and ensure their proper digestion.

Fats: If we do not eat and properly digest sufficient calories, the body will break down first stored fat, then stored protein to supply the energy needed for life. Fats are often a significant source of the dietary calories needed by the body to supply the energy for life, as they have more than twice the energy available for metabolism per unit weight than either carbohydrates or proteins (four calories per gram for protein and carbohydrates, nine calories per gram for fats). Incomplete digestion of fats may result in diarrhea and/or, more seriously, essential fatty acid deficiency. Adequate absorption of essential fatty acids is necessary for healthy skin and optimal permeability in the walls of the cells, allowing nutrients to flow easily into the cells and wastes to flow out.

These days, many health-conscious individuals are eating less fat, protein, and refined sugar and more complex carbohydrates. A diet that consists primarily of cooked food contains few enzymes, since virtually all enzymes are destroyed in cooking. In many cases people are also trying to restrict their caloric intake so that they can lose weight. However, a major stumbling block for most people trying to control their food intake is hunger. We initially experience a feeling of satiety as we chew and swallow our food and receive it into the stomach. Over a longer period of time, we feel satiated as the brain reacts to our body's absorption of all three food categories—protein, carbohydrates, and fats—as they break down. But our failure to digest fats, especially if we are restricting fat intake, reduces or prevents satiety and thus stimulates overeating. Eating effectively alleviates hunger only if the nutrients ingested are also digested and absorbed.

Protein: To maintain health, the human body has developed a complex mechanism for balancing and exchanging proteins and amino acids. Recently many books and diets recommending higher protein intake and lower consumption of carbohydrates have inundated the market. Two of these are Dr. Robert T. Atkins' *Dr. Atkins' New Diet Revolution* and Barry Sears' *The Zone.* While these diets can be beneficial for losing weight and reducing sugar cravings, the body can't utilize these proteins unless it can properly digest them. Improper protein digestion leads to insufficient amino acids in the bloodstream. A shortage of available amino acids will trigger the breakdown of the body's existing protein in order to make up the deficit. When plasma protein levels fall, they are boosted at the expense of other tissues. For this reason, tissue breakdown may occur in the liver or muscle, causing more rapid aging and degeneration.

Eating excessive protein without proper digestion can cause hypoglycemia (low blood sugar), depression, and irritability, since half the protein you digest is converted to sugar.

Protein digestion plays an important part in preventing and eliminating blood clots. In addition, when we do not properly digest protein, this can lead to edema (fluid retention), toxic colon syndrome (a buildup of toxins in the large intestine), constipation, and even colon cancer.

Carbohydrates: Incomplete digestion of carbohydrates causes many problems in the body. These include:

- Breakdown of the proteins in our tissues in order to provide the body with needed energy
- Various forms of intestinal distress, including diarrhea, bloating, and flatulence
- Failure to achieve satiety from the carbohydrates we consume, resulting in overeating and obesity
- Mental symptoms such as depression, mood swings, anger, aggressiveness, violent behavior, and attention deficit hyperactivity disorder
- Spaciness or dizziness that becomes worse when bending
- Insomnia

Another problem resulting from incomplete digestion of carbohydrates is the proliferation of candida, a yeastlike fungus found widely in nature, in the soil, on vegetables and fruits, and in the human body. Candida is frequently present in small quantities in the intestines and in a woman's vagina. When its numbers are few, candida is generally not harmful. But a candida overgrowth, a condition called candidiasis, can become pathogenic and cause allergic reactions throughout the body. These reactions can lead to depression, fatigue, weight gain, anxiety, rashes, headaches, muscle cramping, and sugar cravings.

Insufficient levels of disaccharidase (sugar-digesting) enzymes in the small intestine causes malabsorption of sugars and physical discomfort. The most common and well-known form of this is lactase deficiency. Lactase is the enzyme that digests milk sugar. Lack of this enzyme results in an inability to tolerate milk, producing severe abdominal stress. Another disaccharidase is invertase, which works to break down sucrose (refined table sugar) into glucose and fructose. The prevalence of processed and highly refined foods in the American diet means that we consume a great amount of sucrose, which can contribute to undue digestive stress. It is believed that sucrose intolerance is a contributing factor in many allergies. Taking supplemental doses of disaccharidases augments the breakdown of sugar into glucose molecules, allowing us greater absorption of this energy-giving sugar. Poor sugar digestion can result in strong cravings for sugars and alcohol.

THE ROLE OF FIBER IN DIGESTION

Fiber is an essential component of everyone's diet. There are three general classes of fiber. The first is cellulose, the main structural material in plant cell walls. While the pancreas can manufacture enzymes similar to all of those found in plants, it cannot produce the digestive enzyme cellulase. Since cellulase is not made in the body, it can be obtained only from food sources or enzyme supplements. Another type of fiber is the noncellulose polysaccharides, which include the noncellulose carbohydrates such as pectins, gums, and algae substances. The last is lignin, the only noncarbohydrate type of fiber, which forms the woody part of plants.

The various types of fibers all have different functions. The soluble types of fiber found in beans, barley, vegetables, and fruits protect us against high cholesterol, while the insoluble parts protect against colorectal cancer. Soluble fiber helps lower cholesterol and balance blood sugar better than insoluble fiber. Pectin from fruits binds and eliminates heavy metals from the gastrointestinal tract. And lignin combines with bile acids to help in the excretion of several kinds of waste products.

Fiber also helps food move through the colon more quickly. Maintaining a short transit time between the ingestion of food and the excretion of waste materials is crucial if we are to eliminate toxins from the body as quickly as possible. Colon transit time is usually about fifteen to eighteen hours in people who eat mainly raw, high-fiber foods. In the United States, where the average diet is low in fiber and high in processed foods, excretion usually occurs after two to four days, and it can take up to two weeks among the elderly.

Poor digestion of fiber can result in food allergies, toxic buildup in the colon, bloating and flatulence, and high blood lipids, which contribute to higher cholesterol and triglycerides and the overgrowth of candida or other fungi.

HOW ENZYMES WORK

Enzymes are essential to the precise operation of our bodily functions. They provide the energy that allows all of our physiological and biochemical processes to occur efficiently. Enzymes are so vitally important that I could not even begin to write about the cure for food allergies without an explanation of enzymes and their role in our bodies. In fact, I truly believe food allergies would not exist if we made and/or ingested enough enzymes to completely digest our foods.

Undigested food is the single most prevalent cause of allergic reactions, and a significant number of everyday health problems are linked to poor digestion and resulting allergies. I have seen undigested sugars cause depression, fatigue, bloating, and constipation, and undigested protein cause osteoporosis and menopausal symptoms. A critical aspect of the food allergy cure is to use enzymes to ensure the proper digestion of the foods we eat.

Enzymes perform so many important functions in the body that they are central to most metabolic activity. Enzymes digest food, deliver nutrients, carry away toxic waste, purify the blood, deliver hormones, balance cholesterol and triglyceride levels, feed the brain, build protein into muscle, and feed and fortify the endocrine system. Enzymes also contribute to the healthy functioning of the immune system. White blood cells are especially enzyme-rich, which helps them to digest foreign substances that invade the body.

Other responsibilities of enzymes include:

1. Transforming foods into nutritional molecules for the building of muscles, nerves, bones, and glands
2. Helping to store excess nutrients in muscles or in the liver for future use
3. Helping to pass carbon dioxide, a by-product of normal metabolism, from the lungs

4. Metabolizing iron for utilization in red blood cell production

5. Aiding in blood coagulation

6. Liberating healthful oxygen by decomposing hydrogen peroxide (produced by our immune systems to fight infection)

7. Attacking toxic substances in the body so that they can be eliminated, which is essential to maintaining optimal health

8. Helping convert dietary phosphorus to bone

9. Extracting minerals from food so that they can be fully utilized, for example, magnesium, which is required as a catalyst for many intracellular enzymatic reactions, particularly those relating to carbohydrate metabolism

10. Converting protein, carbohydrates, fats, vitamins, and other nutrients for the body's use

One of the advantages of enzymes is that they can cause a chemical reaction without being destroyed—or even changed—in the process, but our bodies' production of enzymes has limitations. We have a harder time producing enzymes when our bodies must cope with mercury-containing amalgam dental fillings, illnesses such as colds and fevers, pregnancy, stress, strenuous exercise, injuries, and extreme weather conditions. Each enzyme performs a certain amount of work before it becomes exhausted and must be replaced by another. So we must constantly replenish our enzyme supply.

Our bodies are not our only source of enzymes. We also take in enzymes from the foods we eat. Unfortunately, that supply has been seriously diminished. Any form of cooking or processing destroys the enzymes found naturally in food—whether the method involves pasteurization, irradiation, microwaving, or steaming. Our current large-scale agricultural business has caused a drastic reduction of enzymes in our soil due to the use of pesticides and fungicides. Healthy soil should be rich not only in earthworms but in enzymes, vitamins, minerals, and essential microorganisms. Pesticides and fungicides create dead soil, which in turn creates food severely depleted in enzymes.

The enzymes that are available to us are further crippled by inadequate chewing and our high consumption of things such as coffee, pastries concocted of refined flour and sugar, hormone-laden meats, artificial sweeteners, artificial fats, and margarine.

When we do not eat an enzyme-rich diet, we deplete our enzyme potential without replenishing it. This is why taking enzyme supplements and striving to eat a healthier, organic diet well supplied with enzymes is essential. The human body does have the capacity to store the enzymes that we get from food and supplements, which explains the abundance of new enzyme health products on the market and the recommendations from experts that people supplement their diet with raw foods and manufactured food enzymes.

Enzymes can save people's lives by restoring energy and balance, reversing the aging process, turning a dysfunctional digestive system into a healthy one, and strengthening the immune system. In fifteen years of working with enzyme therapy, I have witnessed enormous success with a variety of illnesses. The most noticeable and immediate change in each case has always been in the energy level.

A MIRACULOUS RECOVERY

ᴈᴎ CYNTHIA'S STORY

An excellent example of how enzymes work to cure a variety of problems can be seen in the remarkable recovery of a client named Cynthia. Cynthia, age forty-four, came to me complaining of chronic fatigue, allergies, headaches, occasional colds, frequent sinus infections, and postnasal drip. Since she was an elementary-school teacher, she needed to be active and energetic to keep pace with her students. In addition, Cynthia suffered from severe menstrual and premenstrual symptoms, including weight gain, depression, irritability, sore and swollen breasts, a craving for sweets, painful cramps, and lower back pain.

Cynthia's diagnostic enzyme evaluation exam revealed that she had difficulty digesting and absorbing sugars and fat. Her diet consisted mostly of sugary foods such as fruits and high-carbohydrate bars, with very little protein. Interestingly enough, protein was the one food her body could handle, yet she ate very little of it. The meridian balancing and detoxification examination that I performed on her to determine her organ toxicity revealed moderate liver and lymphatic toxicity. I also discovered calcium and magnesium deficiencies.

Based on these findings, I recommended that Cynthia utilize an enzyme to help her to digest and absorb sugars, a homeopathic liver detoxification remedy, and an enzyme-rich calcium-magnesium formula that not only supplies calcium and magnesium but also provides enzymes to help in the absorption of all trace minerals. Lastly, I gave her an enzyme formula to promote detoxification of the lymphatic system.

The lymphatic system is one of the most important cleansing systems in the body. It is made up of three parts: a vast network of vessels that transport the lymph; a series of nodes throughout the body, primarily in the neck, groin, and armpits, which collect the lymph; and three organs, the tonsils, spleen, and thymus gland, that produce white blood cells called lymphocytes, which are vital to the immune system.

The lymph itself is the fluid found in the space between our cells, which occupies about 18 percent of the body. It contains plasma proteins, foreign particles, and bacteria that accumulate between cells. The purpose of the lymphatic system is to collect the waste products and cellular debris from our tissues and to return them to the blood, where they can be removed. To do this, the lymph flows slowly from all parts of the body toward the chest, where it drains into the bloodstream through two large ducts.

The lymph system becomes particularly active during illnesses such as the flu, when the nodes, especially in the throat area, visibly swell with collected waste products. Congestion in the lymphatic system can result in water retention, sinus congestion, and tiredness.

I also gave Cynthia a protease enzyme formula that helps to digest protein into smaller units called amino acids. In addition to protein from food, it digests organisms that are composed of protein, such as the coating on certain viruses; toxins from dead bacteria and other microorganisms; and certain harmful substances produced at the sites of injury or inflammation. Protease strengthens the immune system, which, among other benefits, can help us more easily fight off bacterial infections. The powerful formula I prescribed for Cynthia enhances systemic balance by helping the body to eliminate toxins in the blood, regulate hormonal effects, and maintain healthy organ function.

Two months on this regimen created remarkable changes in Cynthia's overall health, which she described as miraculous. Her fatigue and headaches completely disappeared, and her premenstrual symptoms were a thing of the past. She has not experienced one sinus infection since she started on the enzymes and detoxification formula.

Although I have treated similar cases, this one was especially significant. Cynthia was sick so often that she was regularly consuming antibiotics. She was so discouraged that she was close to leaving her job as a teacher, and she was increasingly more depressed.

Her recovery was dramatic. Now she describes herself as feeling healthy and normal for the first time in many years. She has plenty of energy, exercises regularly, and enjoys teaching again.

TYPES OF ENZYMES

There are three main categories of enzymes: (1) metabolic enzymes, which we produce within our bodies, (2) digestive enzymes, which our bodies produce also, and (3) food enzymes.

Metabolic enzymes are responsible for running our bodies at the level of the blood, tissues, and organs. They are required for the growth of cells and the repair and maintenance of all the body's organs and tissues. Metabolic enzymes take protein, fat, and carbohydrates and transform them into the proper balance of working cells and tissues. They also remove worn-out material from the cells, keeping them clean and healthy.

Digestive enzymes aid in the digestion of food and the absorption and delivery of nutrients throughout the body. The most commonly known digestive enzymes are secreted from the pancreas into the small intestine. Each enzyme is specific to a particular compound, which it breaks down.

The three most important enzymes for digestion are protease, which digests protein; amylase, which digests carbohydrates; and lipase, which digests fat.

Food enzymes are derived solely from raw fruits, vegetables, and supplemental sources. Like digestive enzymes, they enable our bodies to digest the food we eat by breaking down the various nutrients we consume—proteins, fats, sugars, starches, and fibers—into smaller compounds that the body can absorb. They are absolutely essential in maintaining optimal health.

Overwhelming evidence shows that food enzymes play an important role by predigesting food in the upper stomach. Supplementation with food or vegetarian enzymes is necessary today because so much of the food in a typical American diet is processed or cooked—as much as 85 percent, according to recent studies.

Most food enzymes are essentially destroyed at the temperatures used to cook and process food. Food enzymes are extremely sensitive to temperatures above 118 degrees Fahrenheit. When raw foods are processed or heated in any way, they may lose 100 percent of their enzyme activity and up to 85 percent of their vitamin and mineral content. When we place the full digestive burden on the body, it can become overstressed and vital nutrients may not be assimilated.

Unlike supplemental enzymes of animal origin, plant enzymes work at the level of acidity (pH) found in the upper stomach. Food sits in the upper portion of the stomach for as much as an hour before gastric secretions begin. Although salivary enzymes accomplish a significant amount of digestion, their activity is limited to a pH level above 5.0. Plant enzymes are active in the pH range of 3.0 to 9.0 and can facilitate the utilization of a much larger amount of protein, carbohydrates, and fat before hydrochloric acid is secreted in sufficient amounts to neutralize their activity. Obviously, plant enzymes can play a significant role in improving food nutrient utilization.

Unfortunately, even the raw food we eat might be enzyme-deficient if it was grown in nutrient-lacking soil. In addition, enzyme deterioration begins the moment the food is picked.

To function properly, food enzymes must also work in tandem with the coenzymes of vitamins and minerals. Unlike the enzymes in raw plant foods, coenzymes are not completely destroyed by cooking. But unless the enzymes from raw food are present, the coenzymes in our diet cannot be utilized to their full potential.

For all these reasons, supplementing with enzymes is crucial to achieving a more efficient digestive process and better absorption of our food's nutrients.

When digestion is not properly completed, partially digested proteins putrefy, partially digested carbohydrates ferment, and partially digested fats turn rancid. These toxins then remain in the body, harming the system. For example, toxins in the digestive tract can be absorbed into the blood and deposited as waste in the joints and other soft-tissue areas.

Our digestive processes have first priority on the limited number of internal enzymes available. Metabolic enzymes must be satisfied with whatever is left. When we receive the proper amount of food enzymes from sources outside the body, we do not need to manufacture as many digestive enzymes. This allows us to allocate more of our enzyme potential toward the production of the metabolic enzymes we need for growth, maintenance, and repair.

When we have an enzyme deficiency, however, we develop many health problems. These include digestive disturbances, fatigue, headaches, constipation, gas, heartburn, bloating, colon problems, excess body fat, and problems as serious as cardiovascular disease. Enzyme deficiencies have been linked to premature aging and degenerative diseases as well. In fact, studies have shown that diets deficient in enzymes can cause a 30 percent reduction in life span. Cancer research has discovered that certain enzymes are absent in the blood and urine of many cancer patients. Lack of enzymes and the resulting malabsorption of nutrients can also cause allergic reactions, poor healing of wounds, skin problems, and mood swings.

Enzyme supplements help create more energy, promote faster and easier digestion, and encourage superior nutrient absorption. Our digestive system works best when enzyme supplements assist in setting the nutrients free for the body to absorb and use. Receiving all the nutrients in the food we eat is critical, since these nutrients are needed to build and repair the body's tissue, produce energy, and maintain a strong immune system.

ENZYMES: A KEY TO TREATING HERPES

Research is now suggesting that the herpes simplex virus type II (the type that usually causes genital herpes) may be a prominent factor in transforming normal cells into cancer cells. Hence it is important to avoid flareups of the virus as much as possible. Herpes is an insidious disease. Once it is contracted, the virus cannot be expelled from the body but remains dormant most of the time, usually becoming active under certain circumstances. Most people who have herpes (either type I, which causes cold sores, or type II) know what activates it, but they often have no way of avoiding it. Enzyme therapy can control or eliminate the outbreak.

I have found that the virus is often reactivated when the body becomes weakened through illness, the overgrowth of other viruses, toxicity, physical and digestive stress, hormonal shifts, and fatigue. When these viruses erupt, they penetrate healthy cells and reproduce themselves within those cells. Recent research has found that only a small number of viruses is needed to cripple the immune system to a state of suppression. With enzymes and allergy elimination, I have had success in treating all the different forms of herpes, as well as other kinds of viruses.

✌ JIM'S STORY

Jim, a forty-nine-year-old man, came to see me with chronic cold sores caused by herpes simplex type I. He was referred to me by his wife, a patient I had successfully treated for chronic fatigue. Jim noticed that certain activities—eating certain foods and especially exposing himself to the sun—would activate the herpes. No matter what he did, he could not control it, and he'd struggled with this problem his whole life.

After Jim completed the nutritional and enzyme questionnaire, I performed an enzyme evaluation. The results showed that he was unable to digest fats and proteins and that he had an area of marked dysfunction related to his liver and spleen. I recommended enzymes to facilitate Jim's digestion of protein and fats. I also suggested that he take enzyme supplements containing vitamin C, bioflavonoids, B vitamins, vitamin E, and essential fatty acids. Finally, I told Jim to take an herbal preparation made from milk thistle and barberry bark, to support liver function. All these enzyme preparations are high in protease and supportive of the immune response and spleen function, and are very effective of preventing and clearing herpes outbreaks. It has been two years now since we began treatment, and Jim has not had a recurrence of the cold sores.

Under optimal conditions, the human body is quite capable of producing the enzymes necessary to digest food and allow for the absorption of nutrients. However, with as many as twenty million Americans suffering from various digestive disorders, optimal conditions rarely exist.

After a large meal, many people notice a sudden feeling of sluggishness and energy loss. That is because the body is dealing with an overload of calories and nutrients that it must break down and deliver to the bloodstream. If the food you ate was cooked, then there were no enzymes included to assist in the energy-consuming task of digestion. If you take a digestive enzyme supplement at the beginning of a meal, however, the body is now prepared to handle the new food entering the digestive system. Without this additional supply of enzymes, it may take the body up to sixty minutes to gather the needed enzymes, sometimes even borrowing them from other metabolic processes. (The enzymes designed for digestion of foods are also taken directly before eating.) Supplemental enzymes improve the level of our digestion and help ensure that we attain the maximum level of nutrient absorption.

FOOD AND STRESS

The subject of stress is quite prominent in our current understanding of health and disease. Stress gradually depletes our reserve capacity to deal with extreme challenges to our system. The more reserve capacity our system has, the less likely it is to encounter challenges with which it cannot cope. As our reserve capacity is depleted, however, it becomes more probable that our systems will incur damage because less-extreme circumstances will have a greater effect upon us.

The interplay between stress, reserve capacity, and damage in our bodies can be understood through an analogy to the wear and tear on automobile tires. Driving produces stress on the tire's tread, which gradually removes rubber. This depletes the reserve capacity of the tire, that is, it decreases the thickness of the tread. Bad road surfaces and/or sudden vehicle maneuvers are extreme circumstances that must be handled. As the tire's tread gets thin, there is a reduction in traction, and therefore the chance for structural damage increases. Safe, low-stress driving on well-paved roads minimizes both the rate of tread wear and the chance of encountering extreme conditions.

If most of the diet lacks digestive enzymes, then the body is required to endure either digestive stress or nutritional deficiencies. In the worst-case scenario, both of these circumstances may occur. Systemic stress may occur even after proper digestion and absorption if the nutrients needed by the body are simply not present. Thus a high-stress diet will have one or more of the following characteristics:

- The nutrients ingested are substantially out of balance with the body's metabolic requirements. In other words, there is too little or too much of something.
- The nutrients ingested are not bioavailable because we have an insufficient digestive capacity.
- The foods we ingest cause excessive digestive stress to the body, due to a lack of enzymes in the food.

The results of eating a high-stress diet may include any combination of the following:

- Lack of energy
- Frequent illnesses from a poorly functioning immune system
- Wasting and/or brittleness of bones
- Poor weight control—being over- or underweight
- Indigestion, bloating, gas
- Hormonal imbalances
- Dry or oily skin
- Poor elimination—constipation or frequent loose stools

It is therefore highly desirable to supplement our usual diets, which are primarily composed of cooked and processed foods, with active digestive enzymes, thus reducing the digestive stress on our bodies.

FOOD INTOLERANCES AND DIETARY STRESS

In my practice I see many patients with chronic food intolerances. For example, people can inherit or develop intolerances to proteins, sugars, fibers, complex carbohydrates, or fats. These patients lack the enzymes they need to break down the food they consume. Through enzymatic testing I am able to ascertain which foods a person cannot tolerate and which enzymes they need to take as supplements to restore homeostasis. With the proper enzyme supplements these patients regain the ability to digest their food properly and thoroughly. At the end of this chapter there is a questionnaire similar to one I use in my clinic that will enable you to determine your specific food intolerance.

THERAPEUTIC USE OF ENZYMES

We receive many benefits when we consume food enzymes. These benefits aid in the elimination of the following:

- Heartburn
- Gas
- Headaches

- Bloating
- Colon problems
- Stress
- Fatigue after meals
- Overweight and underweight
- Constipation or loose stools
- Weakened immune system
- Food allergies and hay fever

Some people claim that supplemental enzymes cannot survive the strong acids in the stomach. The manufacturers of these products reply that although these enzymes may disintegrate when mixed with acid in a laboratory test tube, they do not do so in a living human body because stomach acids are mixed with food—buffering them against the strong acidity. Our enzymes continue to digest food in the stomach up to an hour after eating. This is true of the digestive enzymes in our saliva, the enzymes that are present in raw foods, and enzyme supplements that can be taken to promote digestion. Once predigestion has occurred, food enzymes and supplemental enzymes continue to digest protein, carbohydrates, and fat as the stomach becomes more acidic (with the release of hydrochloric acid).

At a certain level of stomach acidity, food and supplemental enzymes are temporarily inactivated. Pepsin, an enzyme secreted by the stomach, continues the digestion of protein in the stomach. Food and supplemental enzymes become active again in the small intestine, aiding the digestive enzymes secreted by the pancreas to complete the digestion of food.

The following are the main enzymes used therapeutically to help restore the body's balance and strengthen the immune system:

Protease: Breaks down protein into amino acids. Works best in the stomach before the acidity of the stomach becomes too high, *so protease supplements are most effective taken at the beginning of a meal or between meals.* After a meal, protease in the digestive tract *continues* to digest the protein in food. Protease in the body tissues and blood helps reduce inflammation and acts on bacteria, viruses, and even cancerous cells.

Amylase: Breaks down complex carbohydrates (starches) into simpler sugars such as dextrin and maltose. Amylase is secreted by the salivary glands in the mouth and by the pancreas into the intestines.

Lipase: Along with bile from the gallbladder, breaks down fats and assists the absorption of fat-soluble vitamins A, D, E, and K. This enzyme can be helpful in losing weight, if dietary habits are also modified.

Cellulase: Breaks down the cellulose found in fruits, vegetables, grains, and seeds. It can increase the nutritional value of fruits and vegetables, but foods high in cellulose must be chewed well to allow cellulase to do its work, preventing the fermentation of starches and the bloating and gas that can result.

Pectinase: Breaks down pectin-rich foods such as citrus fruits, apples, carrots, beets, and tomatoes.

Lactase: Breaks down lactose, the complex sugar in milk products—ideal for lactose-intolerant individuals. BioSET™ allergy elimination treatments are often effective with lactose intolerance. The production of lactase usually decreases with age.

Bromelain: A natural enzyme derived from pineapples; promotes the digestion of plant and animal proteins when taken with a meal. In the body tissues and blood, it can help reduce inflammation, improve circulation, and enhance the immune response.

Papain: An enzyme derived from papaya, which breaks down protein foods and aids protein digestion.

Invertase: Breaks down sucrose, a form of sugar found in many foods, which can contribute to digestive stress if not properly metabolized.

One of my patients' most common complaints has always been "I don't have enough energy." Before I discovered enzymes, there was little I could do to help them. But enzymes changed the situation dramatically.

For the most part, people have low energy because they are not digesting their food properly and therefore cannot benefit from the energy that food provides. The regular consumption of enzyme supplements gives us numerous positive benefits in terms of ongoing general health, including:

- Prevention of toxic waste buildup in the intestines
- More efficient assimilation of fats and proteins in the body
- More comfortable, efficient absorption of nutrients
- More comfortable digestion of large amounts of carbohydrates
- Accelerated digestive process due to catalyzation from enzymes

Some examples of the benefits of having a body that is fully in balance include the following:

- The respiratory and circulatory systems deliver oxygen to cells in balance with their metabolic requirements.
- The urinary system removes waste products and excesses from the blood in balance with the rate at which they enter the blood from other tissues.
- The bone marrow and spleen manufacture new red blood cells in balance with their rate of attrition.
- The digestive glands secrete digestive enzymes in balance with the quantity and composition of food ingested.
- Ingested food provides nutrients in balance with the metabolic requirements of the body.

✑ TRUDY'S STORY

A thirty-five-year-old woman named Trudy came to see me for chronic fatigue and for being overweight. For years she had been plagued with chronic yeast and vaginal infections, bacterial infections, and bloating. Like so many women, she had tried a variety of supplements, alternative treatments, and almost every diet imaginable, with only temporary improvement. Her yeast infections made sexual intimacy difficult, consequently causing stress in her relationship with her husband.

On the enzyme evaluation exam, Trudy showed an inability to digest sugars. Unfortunately, her diet consisted primarily of sugars and carbohydrates, so much of the food she ate was not being digested properly. She also consumed a great deal of alcohol, which has been known to feed yeast infections.

Other laboratory results revealed severe bowel toxicity, which suggested problems with digestion and elimination, and an intestinal toxemia, causing an imbalance in the intestinal flora. Candida infections thrive throughout the system when there is an unbalanced intestinal environment. Her urine, saliva, and blood were severely acidic also, indicating serious digestive dysfunction.

I prescribed Trudy an enzyme to help her digest sugars and an acidophilus formula for intestinal support. Our main goals of helping her to strengthen her immune function and to reduce her chronic vaginal infections were reached within two months. She was very pleased and, to her astonishment, also lost twenty pounds.

✑ MARCUS'S STORY

Marcus, age nine, had become increasingly sick since the age of five with severe food allergies causing stomachaches, headaches, and fatigue. He was frequently out of school with bronchitis and ear infections, and he took repeated courses of antibiotics. Marcus had already undergone numerous blood and urine tests, all of which produced no answers. When Marcus came to see me, I immediately tested him for food allergies. I found that he was highly allergic to grains, such as wheat, oats, and corn. I have found that with children, food allergies are the main cause of illnesses. They weaken the body's immune defense, subjecting the child to chronic infections and fatigue.

(continued)

On that same day I had Marcus's mother, Julie, complete the enzyme evaluation questionnaire. The answers pointed directly to severe sugar intolerance and poor digestion of sugars. Marcus's diet, like that of many children and adults, consisted mainly of refined carbohydrates: cereals, breads, pasta, sodas, and candy bars.

I prescribed an enzyme for digesting sugars, which would help him tolerate grains; a protease enzyme for immune support; and an enzyme formula containing vitamin C, since I detected a deficiency. I also gave him a homeopathic remedy that promoted gentle drainage of the toxins in his body. I recommended that he follow a special diet for sugar-intolerant individuals, and gave his mother strict instructions to eliminate processed foods from his diet.

After one month, Marcus's mother reported great improvement in her son's health. He had regained his vitality and was able to eat grains with no allergic reactions. His stomachaches, headaches, and infections were gone.

A SELF-DIAGNOSTIC ENZYME QUESTIONNAIRE

This questionnaire was created by Dr. Sarah Buchanan and myself and will allow you to evaluate your specific dietary intolerances and then determine the appropriate plant enzyme supplement(s). I recommend everyone take the Digestive Health Formula immediately before meals. Not only will this prepare the way for the mitigation of your food allergies, but it may eliminate some of them immediately. Most important, taking enzyme supplements will help you to gain optimal health and longevity. Enzyme supplements used for prevention or the management of a health condition should be taken between meals (one hour before or two hours after eating).

I have included some recommended food-intolerant diets in Chapter 11, along with some recipes. The recommended diet you require (based on your answers to this questionnaire) reflects your specific foods intolerance at a particular time; your needs may change over time, so I suggest reevaluating yourself every six to twelve months. But I have found that usually one of the specific four diets will consistently meet your needs. I suggest adhering to this diet as closely as possible at least four or five days of the week. These diets, along with the appropriate enzymes, will ensure adequate nutrition and prevent food cravings, weight gain, and fatigue. Usually an individual's assessment will describe one specific food-category intolerance, but some may notice an indication of two or three. If this happens, I suggest that you reassess yourself by taking the questionnaire again and try to be as precise as possible in your answers.

While I do suggest reevaluating yourself periodically, it is not uncommon for a person to need the same enzyme for life. When patients ask me why they need to remain on enzymes permanently, I remind them that if they do not wish to supplement with enzymes, they need to chew each morsel of food at least thirty times so that complete digestion can take place. Anyone who chooses to do this must also remember to eat only uncooked, unprocessed food filled with enzymes and nutrients—which is as important as proper chewing.

FOOD INTOLERANCES AND SENSITIVITIES

The following questions also relate to specific dietary intolerances. If you answer yes to any question, I recommend WellZyme Digestive Health, a multiple-digestive-enzyme formula that suits all the specific intolerances. (See Appendix 1 for more information on the WellZyme formulas.) Following the yes answers is the name of the best diet for that particular intolerance. See Chapter 11 for diet plans and recipes for each type of food intolerance.

1. Do you often feel full over an hour after a meal of average size?
   - ❏ Yes (sugar-intolerant diet)
   - ❏ No

2. Do you experience cramping or bloating immediately after eating despite trying to change the amount of food you eat?
   - ❏ Yes (fat-intolerant diet)
   - ❏ No

3. Do you have difficulty gaining weight or keeping weight on?

❑ Yes (protein-intolerant diet)

❑ No

4. Do you experience abdominal bloating, gas, and an inability to break down fiber-rich foods?

❑ Yes (complex-carbohydrate-intolerant diet or fiber-intolerant diet)

❑ No

5. Do you often experience gas or bloating after eating particular foods?

❑ Meats, soy, or other protein

❑ Yes (protein-intolerant diet)

❑ No

❑ Raw fruits, vegetables, or fiber

❑ Yes (fiber-intolerant diet or complex-carbohydrate-intolerant diet)

❑ No

❑ Simple carbohydrates (breads, sweets, sugars)

❑ Yes (sugar-intolerant diet)

❑ No

❑ Milk or dairy products

❑ Yes (sugar-intolerant diet)

❑ No

❑ Fried foods, butter, or margarine

❑ Yes (fat-intolerant diet)

❑ No

6. Do you ever feel dizzy or emotionally out of sorts after eating certain foods?

❑ Meats, soy, or other protein

❑ Yes (protein-intolerant diet)

❑ No

❑ Raw fruits, vegetables, or fiber

❑ Yes (fiber-intolerant diet)

❑ No

❑ Simple carbohydrates (breads, sweets, sugars)
    ❑ Yes (sugar-intolerant diet)
    ❑ No

❑ Milk or dairy products
    ❑ Yes (sugar-intolerant diet)
    ❑ No

❑ Fried foods, butter, or margarine
    ❑ Yes (fat-intolerant diet)
    ❑ No

7. Do you have frequent bouts with stomach pains or cramping, especially after eating particular foods?

❑ Meats, soy, or other protein
    ❑ Yes (protein-intolerant diet)
    ❑ No

❑ Raw fruits, vegetables, or fiber
    ❑ Yes (fiber-intolerant diet)
    ❑ No

❑ Carbohydrates (breads, sweets, sugars)
    ❑ Yes (sugar-intolerant diet)
    ❑ No

❑ Milk or dairy products
    ❑ Yes (sugar-intolerant diet)
    ❑ No

❑ Fried foods, butter, or margarine
    ❑ Yes (fat-intolerant diet)
    ❑ No

8. Do you crave certain foods?

❑ Sugar (chocolate, candy, cake)
    ❑ Yes (sugar-intolerant diet)
    ❑ No

❑ Protein (meat, chicken, fish, soy)
    ❑ Yes (protein-intolerant diet)
    ❑ No

❑ Fiber (raw fruits and vegetables, bran)

    ❑ Yes (fiber-intolerant diet)

    ❑ No

❑ Carbohydrates (bread)

    ❑ Yes (sugar-intolerant diet)

    ❑ No

❑ Fat (fried foods)

    ❑ Yes (fat-intolerant diet)

    ❑ No

9. Do you often feel a need for laxative assistance in relieving constipation?

    ❑ Yes (sugar-intolerant diet or protein-intolerant diet—compare with other questions for proper selection)

    ❑ No

In the following questions, the number in parentheses following a yes or no answer refers to the WellZyme product appropriate for that symptom or condition. (See page 286 for a list of WellZyme products corresponding to the numbers.)

10. Do you experience an inability to sleep on a regular basis?

    ❑ Yes (15)

    ❑ No

11. Do you feel you sleep enough to maintain your health?

    ❑ Yes

    ❑ No (15)

12. Do you live in a city or environment in which you are exposed to pollutants or factors that may advance the aging process?

    ❑ Yes (10)

    ❑ No

13. Do you currently take a natural-source antioxidant or vitamin supplement?

    ❑ Yes

    ❑ No (10)

14. Do you currently eat five to ten servings of fruits and vegetables a day?
    ❑ Yes
    ❑ No (10)

There isn't really a specific number of enzymes that I recommend. You can take as many as required to suit your needs. While I usually recommend to my patients that they take no more than five enzymes during one period of time, in the past I have used more than five if really needed. The WellZyme product for general digestion is the most significant tool for food allergy prevention. One capsule of a multiple-enzyme product such as Wellzyme's Digestive Health should be taken before all cooked meals.

11

Recipes and Diet Plans

DIET PLANS FOR FOOD INTOLERANCE

- Diet for Sugar Intolerance
- Diet for Complex Carbohydrate Intolerance
- Diet for Fat Intolerance
- Protein Intolerance Diet

There are countless special diets. Each day new ones are being advertised that guarantee weight loss, increased energy, longevity, increased athletic ability and performance, or something else. Many of them are worthwhile for some but not successful for everyone. There is no one diet that works for everyone, because we are all different. Dietary recommendations are individual—that has been my paradigm for twenty-three years. I find that the four different categories of dietary intolerance that people generally fall into are sugar, complex carbohydrates, fat, and protein. The enzyme evaluation questionnaire in Chapter 10 pinpoints the diet for you.

These diets, if followed closely, can aid in weight loss and weight maintenance. For weight loss, restrict grains, breads, and legumes.

DIET FOR SUGAR INTOLERANCE

Individuals who are sugar-intolerant (the highest percentage of the population—almost 80 percent) tend to crave sugar and suffer from depression, malabsorption, bloating, hyperactivity, asthma, chronic constipation, and severe food allergies. They may also exhibit fatigue and have low blood sugar, exhausted adrenal glands, premenstrual syndrome, and allergies. These individuals usually crave sugar. For weight loss, restrict grains, breads, and legumes.

I recommend a diet that includes:

- Liberal quantities of vegetables (see list on the next page), raw or cooked, mineral water, and herbal teas
- Moderate quantities of lipids (fats), plant protein, and animal protein
- Minimal consumption of sugars, fruits, whole grains, and dairy products
- Avoidance of refined grains and sweet vegetables such as carrots and corn
- Limited intake of salt, including soy sauce and other foods that contain large amounts of salt
- Limited intake of alcohol, because in the body it acts as pure sugar, is high in calories, is void of nutrients, weakens and stresses the adrenal glands, and can cause cravings
- Avoidance of all artificial sweeteners and caffeinated beverages

PROTEINS (3–5 SERVINGS PER DAY)

2 egg whites	2 oz skim ricotta cheese	4 oz beef (3 or fewer servings per week)
1 whole egg	4 oz lamb	4 oz poultry
4 oz fish or shellfish	2 oz skim mozzarella cheese	1 oz spirulina or green protein substitute
3 oz tofu		
2 oz low-fat cottage cheese	4 oz soy protein powder	
4 oz veal		

VEGETABLES (UNLIMITED AMOUNTS)

Lettuce (all types)	Endive	Zucchini
Celery	Beans, yellow or	Cabbage
Radishes	green	Cucumbers
Onions	Kale	Jicama
Yellow squash	Bell peppers	Bok choy
Spinach	Sprouts	Escarole
Asparagus	Tomatoes	Okra

VEGETABLES (3–4 SERVINGS PER WEEK)

4 oz cabbage	4 oz carrots	4 oz peas
1 small artichoke	4 oz sweet potatoes	4 oz yams
4 oz potatoes	4 oz pumpkin	4 oz corn

FRUITS (2 SERVINGS PER DAY)

1 apple	1 pear	¾ c berries
1 peach	2 plums	10 cherries
2 medium apricots	10 grapes	2 prunes
½ c fresh pineapple	1 c watermelon	2 small tangerines
1 nectarine	½ cantaloupe	

FRUITS (3–4 SERVINGS PER WEEK)

½ banana	1½ dates	8 oz fruit juice
½ mango	1 c papaya	½ c cranberries
1½ dried figs	½ c raisins	

COMPLEX CARBOHYDRATES: LEGUMES AND GRAINS (2 SERVINGS PER DAY)

⅓ c cooked lentils

½ c cooked wild rice

1 rice cake

½ c cooked grits

1 (6-inch) corn
   tortilla

½ c cooked millet

½ c cooked brown
   rice

½ c cooked quinoa

½ c cereal (cold
   breakfast cereal
   with no
   preservatives)

½ c cooked artichoke
   pasta

½ oz tortilla chips

½ pita bread

½ c cooked spelt

½ c kamut (cooked)

½ c granola

2 c popped
   popcorn

⅓ c cooked beans

FATS (2 SERVINGS PER DAY)

7 almonds or
   ½ tsp almond
   butter

⅓ tsp canola oil

⅓ tsp olive oil

3 olives

½ tbsp avocado

½ tbsp tahini

1 tsp olive-oil-and-
   vinegar dressing

6 peanuts

FATS (3–4 SERVINGS PER WEEK)

1 tsp mayonnaise

⅓ tsp soybean oil

½ tsp Brazil nuts

⅓ tsp butter

1 tsp cream
   cheese

⅓ tsp lard

½ tbsp peanut
   butter

½ tsp sesame oil

½ tsp walnuts

2 tsp bacon bits

½ tbsp cream

½ tbsp low-fat sour
   cream

⅓ tsp margarine

RECIPES FOR SUGAR-INTOLERANT DIET

FRUIT SLUSHY

Makes 1–2 servings

> *4 oz soy protein powder*
> *1 fruit of choice*
> *6 oz water*
> *$^1/_2$ c ice*

Blend ingredients well.

SKILLET EGGPLANT AND TOFU PASTA

Makes 2 servings

> *$^2/_3$ tsp olive oil*
> *2 c diced pared eggplant*
> *$^1/_4$ c each diced onion, diced red bell pepper, and quartered mushrooms*
> *3 oz diced tofu*
> *1 small garlic clove, minced*
> *1 c canned crushed tomatoes*
> *2 tsp chopped fresh basil*
> *$^1/_8$ tsp each oregano leaves and pepper*
> *1 c cooked small whole-wheat macaroni shells*
> *3 oz shredded mozzarella*

In 9- or 10-inch nonstick skillet heat oil over medium high heat; add eggplant and cook, stirring occasionally, until slightly softened, about 5 minutes. Add onion, bell pepper, tomatoes, basil, oregano, pepper, mushrooms, tofu, and garlic. Increase heat to high; cover and cook, stirring occasionally, until vegetables are tender-crisp, about 5 minutes. Add macaroni, stirring to combine; continue simmering 5 minutes longer. Serve sprinkled with mozzarella cheese.

NO-SUGAR-ADDED TOFU SMOOTHIE

Makes 1–2 servings

> *3 oz silken tofu*
> *1 c berries, any type*
> *6 oz water*
> *½ c of ice*

Blend ingredients well.

STUFFED ZUCCHINI

Makes 4 servings

> *4 medium-sized zucchini (about 7 inches long), minced*
> *2 tsp olive oil*
> *1½ c minced onion*
> *½ lb mushrooms, minced*
> *6 cloves garlic, minced*
> *1½ c cooked brown rice*
> *25 almonds, finely minced (or ground)*
> *3 tbsp lemon juice*
> *Black pepper and cayenne, to taste*
> *Small handfuls of freshly minced herbs, if available (parsley, basil, thyme, dill, chives, marjoram)*

Cut the zucchini lengthwise down the middle. Use a spoon to scoop out the insides, leaving a canoe with a ¼-inch shell. Finely mince the insides; set the canoes aside. Heat the olive oil in a medium-sized skillet. Add onion and sauté over medium heat 5 to 8 minutes, or until the onion is soft.

Add minced zucchini and mushrooms and sauté another 8 to 10 minutes. Add the garlic during the last few minutes.

Place rice and almonds in a bowl. Stir in the zucchini-mushroom mixture and lemon juice and mix well. Season to taste with black pepper, cayenne, and optional fresh herbs. Fill the zucchini shells and bake at 350° for 30 to 40 minutes, or until heated through. Serve hot.

LITE BITE DINNER

4 oz grilled skinless chicken breast with 3 olives

1 cucumber, sliced, mixed with 1 c low-fat yogurt and 1 tsp dried dill

TABOULI

Makes 6 servings

1 c dry bulgur

1¹/₂ c boiling water

¹/₄ c fresh lemon juice

2 tsp olive oil

2 cloves garlic, crushed

Black pepper, to taste

4 scallions, finely minced

1 packed c minced parsley

10 to 15 fresh mint leaves, minced

2 medium ripe tomatoes, diced

1 medium bell pepper, diced

Combine bulgur and boiling water in a bowl. Cover and let stand until the bulgur is tender (20 to 30 minutes, minimum).

Add lemon juice, olive oil, garlic, and black pepper, and mix thoroughly. Cover tightly and refrigerate until about 30 minutes before serving.

About 30 minutes before serving, stir in remaining ingredients and mix well. Serve cold.

SUGAR-INTOLERANT DIET—7-DAY SAMPLE PLAN

MONDAY

BREAKFAST

4 oz soy protein powder, mixed with ¹/₂ c cooked oatmeal

LUNCH

> 4 oz turkey breast rolled into 1 corn tortilla, filled with kale and spinach, with 1 tsp mayonnaise

SNACK

> 10 grapes
> $\frac{1}{2}$ c low-fat yogurt

DINNER

> 2 c grilled mixed zucchini, squash, and tomatoes, with $\frac{1}{3}$ tsp canola oil, topped with 2 oz mozzarella, melted

SNACK

> Fruit Slushy with peaches

TUESDAY

BREAKFAST

> $\frac{1}{2}$ waffle
> 2 egg whites, prepared with cooking spray

LUNCH

> 4 oz grilled salmon
> $\frac{1}{2}$ c pasta
> 1 c grilled mixed bell pepper, tomatoes, and onion, with $\frac{1}{3}$ tsp olive oil

SNACK

> 1 pear
> 1 oz mozzarella

DINNER

> 4 oz lean beef
> Tabouli, 1 serving
> 1 c grilled mushrooms, with $\frac{1}{3}$ tsp olive oil

SNACK

> $^1/_2$ honeydew melon
> 2 egg whites, poached or prepared with cooking spray

WEDNESDAY

BREAKFAST

> $^1/_2$ whole-wheat pita topped with tomato slices and 2 oz mozzarella

LUNCH

> Spinach salad topped with 4 oz grilled chicken breast, $^1/_2$ mango, and
> $^1/_3$ tsp peanut oil

DINNER

> 4 oz lamb
> $^1/_2$ c spelt pasta
> Tossed salad with 1 tsp oil-and-vinegar dressing

SNACK

> $^1/_2$ c cantaloupe
> 2 oz low-fat cottage cheese

THURSDAY

BREAKFAST

> 2 oz low-fat cottage cheese
> 1 rice cake

LUNCH

> Skillet Eggplant and Tofu Pasta, 1 serving

SNACK

> *2 apricots*
> *¹/₂ c low-fat yogurt*

DINNER

> *4 oz grilled skinless chicken breast*
> *1 small sweet potato, with ¹/₃ tsp butter and dash cinnamon*
> *1 c cauliflower with ¹/₃ tsp butter*

SNACK

> *2 plums*
> *¹/₂ c low-fat yogurt*

FRIDAY

BREAKFAST

> *No-Sugar-Added Tofu Smoothie*

LUNCH

> *4 oz grilled chicken breast in ¹/₂ whole-wheat pita with spinach leaves, bok choy, and ¹/₂ tsp walnuts*

SNACK

> *7 almonds*

DINNER

> *4 oz tuna, grilled*
> *Stuffed Zucchini, 1 serving*

SNACK

> *1 c berries*
> *2 oz low-fat cottage cheese*

SATURDAY

BREAKFAST

>1 c low-fat yogurt
>1/2 c granola with raisins

LUNCH

>4 oz grilled fish
>4 oz peas
>1 c grilled mixed mushrooms and onions, with 1/3 tsp olive oil

SNACK

>1 apple
>1 oz mozzarella

DINNER

>4 oz veal
>1 c grilled mixed okra, bell pepper, and onion, with 1/3 tsp canola oil
>1/2 c brown rice

SNACK

>10 peanuts

SUNDAY

BREAKFAST

>1 egg plus 2 egg whites, prepared with cooking spray
>1/2 banana

LUNCH

>4 oz ground beef, very lean
>1 whole-wheat bun
>Lettuce, tomato, onion, mustard

SNACK

Fruit Slushy prepared with nectarine

DINNER

Lite Bite Dinner

SNACK

$^1/_2$ c pineapple
$^1/_2$ c low-fat yogurt

DIET FOR COMPLEX CARBOHYDRATE AND FIBER INTOLERANCE

Individuals who are complex-carbohydrate- and fiber-intolerant usually crave fatty foods and tend toward an irritable bowel. They may experience gas after eating complex carbohydrates and other high-fiber foods such as whole grains, raw vegetables, and beans. The increased gas may occur immediately or sometimes two to three hours after a meal. Many of these people can also be sugar-intolerant as well. For such cases, I recommend the sugar-intolerant diet with the use of an enzyme supplement such as WellZymes' Digestive Health formula *before* and *after* meals. For individuals who are complex-carbohydrate-intolerant, I recommend a diet that includes:

- Restricted grains, breads, and legumes, especially if weight loss is an issue
- Liberal quantities of protein, certain cooked vegetables (see list below), mineral water, and selected herbal teas
- Moderate quantities of fats, plant protein, fruits, and refined carbohydrates
- Minimal consumption of high-fiber foods such as whole grains, nuts, seeds, raw vegetables, and vegetables with seeds
- Limited intake of salt, including soy sauce and other foods that contain large amounts of salt

- Limited intake of alcohol, because in the body it acts as pure sugar, is high in calories, is void of nutrients, and can cause cravings
- Avoidance of all artificial sweeteners and caffeinated beverages

PROTEINS (2–3 SERVINGS PER DAY)

2 egg whites	1 c low-fat or nonfat	4 oz veal
1 whole egg	yogurt	4 oz beef (3 servings
2 oz skim	2 oz low-fat cottage	or less per week)
mozzarella	cheese	3 oz tofu
4 oz soy protein	2 oz skim ricotta	4 oz lamb
powder	1 oz spirulina or	
4 oz fish, shellfish,	green protein	
poultry	substitute	

VEGETABLES (UNLIMITED AMOUNTS)

Cooked cauliflower	Cooked zucchini	Spinach
Cooked onions	Cooked mushrooms	Escarole
Cooked yellow	Cooked artichokes	Kale
squash	Celery	Cabbage
Cooked yellow or	Lettuce (all types)	Jicama
green beans	Onions	Bok choy
Cooked eggplant	Radishes	
Cooked okra	Endives	

VEGETABLES (3–4 SERVINGS PER WEEK)

4 oz sweet peas	4 oz cooked yam	4 oz cooked
4 oz cooked carrots	4 oz cooked sweet	pumpkin
4 oz cooked corn	potatoes	
4 oz cooked potatoes		

VEGETABLES TO AVOID

Tomatoes	Sprouts	Cucumber

FRUITS (2 SERVINGS PER DAY)

1 apple	Fruit juices diluted	1 c berries
1 peach	half and half	½ c fresh
2 apricots	with water	pineapple
¼ honeydrew	1 pear	1 c papaya
10 cherries	1 c grapes	
1 nectarine	2 plums	

FRUITS (3–4 SERVINGS PER WEEK)

1½ c dried figs	½ c cantaloupe	½ c cranberries
1½ c dates	½ banana	
1 c watermelon	½ c raisins	

COMPLEX CARBOHYDRATES: LEGUMES AND GRAINS (1–2 SERVINGS PER DAY)

1 slice whole-grain bread	1 corn tortilla	½ English muffin
½ c cooked bulgur	½ c cooked white rice	½ waffle
½ c cooked quinoa	½ c cooked brown rice	½ pita
½ c cooked pasta		½ c cooked spelt or kamut
⅓ c cooked beans	½ c cooked oatmeal	
1 rice cake	¼ bagel	

AVOID

Popcorn	Tortilla chips	Granola

FATS (1–2 SERVINGS PER DAY)

⅓ tsp canola oil	½ tbsp avocado oil	1 tsp olive-oil-and-vinegar dressing
⅓ tsp olive oil	½ tbsp tahini	
⅓ tsp peanut oil		

FATS (3–4 SERVINGS PER WEEK)

1 tsp mayonnaise	⅓ tsp lard	½ tbsp low-fat
⅓ tsp soybean oil	2 tsp sesame oil	sour cream
⅓ tsp butter	2 tsp bacon bits	⅓ tsp margarine
1 tsp cream cheese	½ tbsp cream	

AVOID

Nuts   Seeds

RECIPES FOR COMPLEX-CARBOHYDRATE-INTOLERANCE DIET

QUINOA AND BULGUR PILAF

Makes 4 servings

$^1/_2$ c bulgur
$^1/_2$ c quinoa
1 tbsp olive oil
1 c sliced carrots
$^1/_2$ c diced zucchini
$^1/_2$ c diced squash
6 green onions
1 c sliced mushrooms
12 oz tofu, diced
6 cloves garlic, minced
$^3/_4$ tsp dried basil
$^1/_2$ tsp oregano
$^1/_2$ tsp dried thyme
$^1/_2$ tsp black pepper

Cook bulgur and quinoa as package directions suggest.

Heat a large skillet and add olive oil. Sauté carrots, zucchini, and squash. Add green onions, mushrooms, tofu and cook until tender. Add garlic, herbs, and pepper and sauté an additional 5 minutes. Combine cooked grains with sautéed vegetables and serve.

CHILLED VEGETABLE-YOGURT SALAD

Makes 4 servings

> *1 c grated cauliflower*
> *1 c grated squash*
> *1 c grated zucchini*
> *2 c water*
> *2 c low-fat yogurt*
> *1 small clove garlic, minced*
> *1 tsp dried dill*
> *Minced fresh mint and chives*

Combine grated vegetables, water, yogurt, garlic, and dill in a bowl. Stir until well blended and chill until very cold. Serve topped with finely minced fresh mint and chives.

WILTED SPINACH SALAD

Makes 2 servings

> *6 oz chicken breast*
> *2 egg whites*
> *Cooking spray*
> *²/₃ tsp olive oil*
> *2 cloves garlic, minced*
> *12 oz spinach*
> *Black pepper*

Bake chicken breast until done; slice and set aside. Scramble egg whites using nonstick cooking spray; crumble and set aside. Heat olive oil and add garlic. Sauté until garlic is opaque. Add spinach to oil and garlic and cook for about 2 minutes, until spinach is wilted. Add chicken breast and egg whites to spinach and sauté for an additional minute. Season with black pepper to taste. Remove from heat and serve.

SPIRULINA SALAD

Makes 1 serving

> 1 oz spirulina
> 1 boiled egg, sliced
> 1 apple, chopped
> Bok choy, torn
> Endive, torn
> Escarole, torn
> ½ tsp peanut oil

Arrange first three ingredients on top of next three ingredients. Top with peanut oil.

GARLICKY STEAMED SUMMER VEGETABLES

Makes 4 servings

> Black pepper, to taste
> ½ lb green beans, trimmed and cut
> 1 c mushrooms, sliced
> 1 c cauliflower, chopped
> 1 medium carrot, diced
> 1 small zucchini, diced
> 1 small squash, diced
> Small bunch spinach, chopped
> 3–4 cloves garlic
> ⅔ tsp olive oil
> Fresh basil, dill, parsley, and/or chives

Steam the vegetables until just tender in the following groupings: green beans; mushrooms, cauliflower, carrots; zucchini, squash, spinach. Set the veggies aside. Sauté garlic in oil for 2 minutes and stir in the steamed vegetables. Season with basil, dill, parsley, and/or chives.

TOFU SPINACH DIP

Makes 4 servings

> 10-oz package frozen spinach
> 12 oz firm tofu, crumbled
> 8-oz can water chestnuts, chopped coarsely
> ²/₃ c green onions, chopped
> ¹/₂ c light mayonnaise
> ¹/₂ c light sour cream

Thaw the spinach, squeeze dry, and chop finely. Stir all ingredients together in a large bowl until blended. Cover; chill 2 hours. Stir before serving.

PASTA WITH SHRIMP AND ARTICHOKE

Makes 2 servings

> 1 c dry pasta such as ziti, penne, or shells
> 1 c artichoke hearts, no salt added
> 1 clove garlic, minced
> ¹/₂ c water
> ²/₃ tsp canola oil
> 8 oz cooked shrimp

Cook pasta according to directions on the box. Put the artichokes, garlic, and water in a large nonstick skillet. Cover, bring to a boil, and let simmer for about 2 minutes. Add the oil and shrimp; heat through. Add the drained pasta; toss well.

TOFU STIR-FRY

Makes 2 servings

> ¹/₃ tsp olive oil
> 1 c fresh mushrooms
> 1 medium onion, chopped
> 1 medium zucchini, sliced
> 1 medium yellow squash, sliced

> *3 oz tofu*
> *¹/₂ tsp cayenne pepper*
> *¹/₂ tsp curry powder*
> *¹/₂ tsp black pepper*
> *¹/₂ c cooked rice*

Heat olive oil in skillet. Add vegetables and tofu. Add cayenne, curry, and black pepper. Stir well and cook until tender. Serve over rice.

VEGGIE LASAGNA

Makes 4 servings

> *1 large zucchini*
> *1 large squash*
> *1 eggplant*
> *2 oz skim ricotta*
> *2 Portobello mushrooms*
> *Cooking spray*

Peel zucchini, squash, and eggplant. Slice all vegetables thickly. Spray baking sheet with cooking spray, and roast vegetables in oven until golden brown (5–10 minutes).

Layer the mushrooms across the bottom of a 9-inch-square casserole dish coated with cooking spray. Sprinkle half of the ricotta over the mushrooms. Next, layer the zucchini and squash, then the rest of the ricotta, followed by the eggplant on top. Bake at 350° for 30 minutes, until vegetables are tender.

COMPLEX-CARBOHYDRATE-INTOLERANT DIET — 7-DAY SAMPLE PLAN

MONDAY

BREAKFAST

> *1 egg plus 2 egg whites, scrambled*
> *¹/₂ c cooked oatmeal*

LUNCH

> *4 oz grilled fish*
> *Cooked Quinoa and Bulgur Pilaf, 1 serving*

SNACK

> *1 c grapes*

DINNER

> *4 oz lamb*
> *1 c Vegetable-Yogurt Salad*
> *4 oz cooked carrots*
> *1 c steamed cabbage*

SNACK

> *1 nectarine*

TUESDAY

BREAKFAST

> *Smoothie (blend 4 oz soy protein powder, 1 c berries, $^1/_2$ c water, and*
>   *$^1/_2$ c of ice)*

LUNCH

> *4 oz grilled chicken on a bed of Wilted Spinach Salad, topped with*
>   *balsamic vinegar*
> *$^1/_2$ pita bread, toasted*

SNACK

> *2 oz part-skim mozzarella*

DINNER

> *4 oz grilled salmon with lemon-pepper seasoning*
> *1 c grilled mixed okra and onions, with $^1/_3$ tsp olive oil*
> *$^1/_3$ c cooked black beans*

SNACK

1 pear

WEDNESDAY

BREAKFAST

1 c low-fat yogurt
¹/₄ bagel, toasted, with spray butter

LUNCH

4 oz veal
1 c roasted eggplant
¹/₂ c cooked brown rice

SNACK

¹/₂ c fresh pineapple
2 oz low-fat cottage cheese

DINNER

Spirulina Salad, 1 serving

THURSDAY

BREAKFAST

2 oz part-skim mozzarella
¹/₂ English muffin

LUNCH

4 oz grilled tuna with salt-free Cajun seasoning
1 c Garlicky Steamed Summer Vegetables
1 slice whole-grain bread, toasted, with spray butter
1 c papaya chunks

SNACK

Lots of celery, dipped into 3 oz Tofu and Spinach Dip

DINNER

4 oz baked chicken breast
4 oz sweet potato, with dash cinnamon and $\frac{1}{2}$ tsp butter
1 c steamed spinach with artichokes

SNACK

$\frac{1}{2}$ banana
1 c low-fat yogurt

FRIDAY

BREAKFAST

1 egg, hard-boiled or prepared with cooking spray
1 slice whole-grain bread

LUNCH

$\frac{1}{2}$ artichoke with 4 oz cooked shrimp over $\frac{1}{2}$ c cooked pasta with $\frac{1}{3}$ tsp
   canola oil
Large spinach salad topped with balsamic vinegar

SNACK

4 oz soy protein powder mixed with 4 oz juice and 4 oz water, blended
   with ice

DINNER

Tofu Stir-Fry

SATURDAY

BREAKFAST

> *2 oz low-fat cottage cheese*
> *1 c berries*

LUNCH

> *1 c low-fat yogurt*
> *2 rice cakes*
> *1 plum*

SNACK

> *1 apricot*

DINNER

> *4 oz grilled tenderloin or sirloin*
> *4 oz baked potato with ¹/₃ tbsp lite sour cream*
> *Large salad with lettuce, onions, celery, radishes, and balsamic vinegar*

SNACK

> *¹/₄ c honeydew*

SUNDAY

BREAKFAST

> *4 oz soy protein powder blended with 8 oz juice and ice*

LUNCH

> *Grilled cheese sandwich (2 oz part-skim mozzarella on 2 slices whole-grain bread, grilled with ¹/₃ tsp butter)*
> *Large salad with lettuce, spinach, kale, and 1 tsp olive-oil-and-vinegar dressing*

SNACK

1 hard-boiled egg

DINNER

Veggie Lasagna, 1 serving

DIET FOR FAT INTOLERANCE

Individuals who are fat-intolerant may be deficient in the essential fatty acids because of their problems digesting and absorbing fats. They may also demonstrate symptoms of thyroid imbalance such as dry skin or eczema; weight loss or weight gain; fatigue; cold hands and feet; hair loss; diminished growth of nails, skin, and hair; menstrual irregularities; and infertility. These individuals tend to crave sugars and salt and are also prone to liver and gallbladder problems.

For these individuals, I recommend a diet that includes:

- Liberal quantities of vegetables (raw or cooked without fat or salt–see list on next page), fruits, legumes, vegetable protein, mineral water, vegetable juices, fruit juices, and selected herbal teas
- Moderate quantities of higher-fat protein sources such as seafood, low-fat dairy products, whole grains (see list on page 259 under complex carbohydrates) and starchy vegetables such as potatoes, yams, and winter squash
- Avoidance or minimal consumption of animal fats, tropical oils, hydrogenated oils, butter, cocoa butter (found in chocolate), margarine, mayonnaise, shortening, meats, whole-milk dairy products, nuts, egg yolks, fried foods, nondairy creamers, and refined grains
- Use sparingly: olive oil, canola oil, avocado oil, sesame oil, peanut oil, corn oil, cottonseed oil, sunflower oil, soybean oil, safflower oil, and walnut oil (1 tsp 1–2 times per day)
- Limited intake of olives and avocadoes

- Limited intake of salt, including soy sauce and other foods that contain large amounts of salt
- Limited intake of alcohol, because it is irritating to the liver, can cause cravings, acts as pure sugar in the body, is high in calories, and is void of nutrients
- Avoidance of nuts, all nut butters, cream cheese, sour cream, bacon, artificial sweeteners, and caffeinated beverages

For weight loss, limit red meat, dairy products, kidney and lima beans, and wheat, and use only nonfat or low-fat dairy products.

PROTEINS (2 SERVINGS PER DAY)

2 egg whites	2 oz farmer	3 oz tofu
3 oz fish or shellfish	cheese	3 oz lean beef (no
3 oz lean poultry	2 oz skim ricotta	more than 3
2 oz nonfat	cheese	times per week)
powdered milk	3 oz soy cheese	3 oz lean lamb (no
2 oz low-fat or	6 oz nonfat or	more than 3
nonfat cottage	low-fat yogurt	times per week)
cheese	⅓ c soybeans	

VEGETABLES: UNLIMITED

Beets	Radishes	Kale
Broccoli	Sprouts	Lettuce
Cauliflower	Water chestnuts	Okra
Cucumbers	Green or yellow	Parsley
Endives	beans	Rutabagas
Jicama	Bok choy	Squash
Leeks	Celery	Spinach
Onions	Escarole	Watercress

VEGETABLES (3–4 SERVINGS PER WEEK)

Artichokes	Sweet peas	Corn
Mushrooms	Potatoes	Sweet potatoes
Olives	Yams	Pumpkins
Peppers	Carrots	

COMPLEX CARBOHYDRATES: LEGUMES AND GRAINS (2–3 SERVINGS PER DAY)

⅓ c cooked dried beans	½ c cooked amaranth	1 6-inch corn tortilla
⅓ c cooked brown rice	½ c cooked buckwheat	½ c cooked oatmeal
⅓ c cooked wild rice	½ c cooked millet	½ c cooked steel-cut oats
1 rice cake	½ c cooked kamut	
½ c cooked lentils	½ c cooked spelt	
½ c cooked barley	½ c cooked grits	

FRUITS (3 SERVINGS PER DAY)

1 small apple	¼ melon (casaba,	4 medium fresh apricots
1½ dried figs	Christmas,	
½ grapefruit	crenshaw,	¾ c berries
1 lemon	musk,	12 cherries
10 grapes	watermelon,	2½ medium dates
½ mango	honeydew)	1 peach
1 small pear	1¼ c strawberries	2 medium prunes
2 plums		

RECIPES FOR FAT-INTOLERANT DIET

CHICKEN WITH MUSHROOMS AND ARTICHOKES

Makes 4 servings

> 4 boneless, skinless, 3 oz chicken breasts
> Cooking spray
> 8 oz fresh mushrooms
> 8 oz artichoke hearts, no salt added
> 1 lemon

Grill the chicken breasts without adding any oil or fat. Spray skillet with cooking spray. Sauté mushrooms and artichoke hearts until tender. Squeeze juice of a fresh lemon onto mushrooms and artichoke hearts, and serve over grilled chicken breast.

BREAKFAST SMOOTHIE

Makes 2 servings

> 3 oz soft tofu
> $1^1/_4$ c strawberries
> 6 oz water
> 1 scoop of ice

Blend well.

GRILLED LEMON PEPPER SALMON

Makes 2 servings

> 4 oz salmon
> Cooking spray
> 1 tsp black pepper
> 1 lemon

Grill salmon, using cooking spray to prevent sticking. Sprinkle with black pepper and squeeze fresh lemon onto salmon.

CUCUMBER DIP

1 cucumber, finely chopped
1 celery stalk, finely chopped
¹/₄ c fresh leeks, finely chopped
2 oz nonfat yogurt

Combine cucumber, celery, and leeks in a bowl. Add yogurt and mix well.

SHRIMP AND JICAMA

Makes 2 servings

1 jicama
4 oz medium shrimp, peeled and deveined
1 tbsp salt-free Cajun seasoning
Cooking spray

Peel jicama and slice into thick or thin slices, depending on preference. Sprinkle both shrimp and jicama with salt-free Cajun seasoning. Grill or roast shrimp and jicama with cooking spray until shrimp are thoroughly cooked.

BAKED TORTILLA CHIPS

1 tortilla
Cooking spray
1 tbsp salt-free Cajun seasoning

Slice tortillas into 8 triangles. Spray tortillas with cooking spray and sprinkle with salt-free Cajun seasoning. Bake at 350° until crispy.

ROASTED EGGPLANT

Makes 4 servings

1 large eggplant
Cooking spray
¹/₂ tsp cayenne pepper

$^1/_2$ *tsp dried thyme*

1 lemon

Slice eggplant into thick slices. Spray with cooking spray and sprinkle with cayenne and thyme. Squeeze fresh lemon over eggplant. Roast in 350° oven until lightly browned.

STIR FRY

Makes 4 servings

1 large zucchini or crookneck squash

1 large red onion

1 large red pepper

1 tsp garlic granules

1 tsp chili powder

Cooking spray

Cut squash into 1-inch chunks. Do the same with onion and bell pepper. Place chunks into a large bowl. Sprinkle with remaining ingredients. Sauté with cooking spray for 10 minutes or until tender when pierced with fork.

FAT-INTOLERANT DIET — 7-DAY SAMPLE PLAN

MONDAY

BREAKFAST

2 egg whites, prepared with cooking spray

$^1/_2$ *c grits*

1 small apple

LUNCH

6 oz nonfat yogurt

10 grapes

$^1/_2$ *c raw carrots*

1 rice cake

SNACK

> *1 slice whole-grain bread, toasted, with spray butter*

DINNER

> *3 oz sirloin or tenderloin steak*
> *1 c steamed cabbage with salt-free Cajun seasoning*
> *$^1/_3$ c cooked lentils*

TUESDAY

BREAKFAST

> *2 oz nonfat cottage cheese*
> *$^1/_2$ banana*
> *1 slice whole-grain bread*

LUNCH

> *Chicken Topped with Mushrooms and Artichokes*
> *$^1/_3$ c wild rice*
> *Salad*

SNACK

> *2 medium prunes*

DINNER

> *3 oz tofu*
> *Sprouts, water chestnuts, celery, and green beans rolled into 2 corn*
>   *tortillas*

SNACK

> *$^3/_4$ c berries*

WEDNESDAY

BREAKFAST

Breakfast Smoothie
¹/₂ bagel

LUNCH

4 oz Lemon Pepper Salmon
4–6 oz grilled or steamed broccoli and cauliflower, with lemon
²/₃ c cooked navy beans

SNACK

1 medium apple

DINNER

3 oz grilled chicken breast, skinless
1 c beets
Cucumber Salad with Celery and Leeks
¹/₂ pita, toasted

SNACK

2 plums

THURSDAY

BREAKFAST

6 oz nonfat yogurt
³/₄ c berries
1 slice whole-grain bread

LUNCH

3 oz lean beef (sirloin, tenderloin, round)
Small baked potato, with spray butter and salt and pepper

Green salad, with lemon juice
$^1/_3$ c cooked lentils

SNACK

2 small tangerines

DINNER

3 oz lean lamb
1 c mixed okra and onions sautéed in cooking spray, seasoned with red and
    black pepper
1 c cooked whole-wheat pasta

SNACK

$^1/_2$ mango

FRIDAY

BREAKFAST

$^1/_2$ c cooked oatmeal mixed with 2 oz nonfat dry milk powder
1 peach

LUNCH

Shrimp and Jicama, 1 serving, over $^1/_2$ c brown rice
Tossed spinach salad, with balsamic vinegar

SNACK

$^1/_3$ cantaloupe

DINNER

3 oz grilled fish with salt-free Cajun seasoning
Small sweet potato, with spray butter and cinnamon
1 c steamed broccoli
1 slice whole-wheat bread

SNACK

> 1 oz or 14 baked tortilla chips
> ½ pita, toasted

SATURDAY

BREAKFAST

> ½ c cooked barley with 2 medium prunes
> 2 egg whites, prepared with cooking spray

LUNCH

> 3 oz grilled chicken breast
> Roasted Eggplant, 1 serving
> ⅓ c cooked pinto beans

SNACK

> ½ grapefruit

DINNER

> Stir Fry, 1 serving, served over ⅔ c wild rice

SNACK

> 1¼ c strawberries, sweetened with stevia (natural sweetener)

SUNDAY

BREAKFAST

> 1 small whole-wheat bagel
> 2 oz nonfat cottage cheese
> ¾ c fresh pineapple

LUNCH

Tossed salad topped with 3 oz tuna and fresh lemon juice
¹/₂ whole-wheat pita

SNACK

¹/₂ banana

DINNER

3 oz grilled chicken breast, skinless
1 c green beans and mushrooms, steamed
¹/₂ c noodles

SNACK

1 orange

PROTEIN-INTOLERANT DIET

Individuals who are protein-intolerant usually crave sugar and tend to experience anxiety, poor calcium absorption, and hypoglycemia. They feel sluggish when eating animal protein and can experience fluid retention and constipation. Protein-intolerant individuals crave sugars and protein.

A protein-intolerant diet should consist of:

- Liberal quantities of vegetables (raw or cooked without fat or salt—see list on next page), fruits, mineral water, hot grain beverages, vegetable juices, fruit juices, and selected herbal teas
- Moderate quantities of whole grains (see list on page 269) and starchy vegetables such as potatoes, yams, and winter squash
- Minimal consumption of all proteins, legumes, animal fats, tropical oils, hydrogenated vegetable oils, fried foods, whole-milk dairy products, coconut, macadamia nuts
- Limited intake of salt, including soy sauce and other foods that contain large amounts of salt

- Limited intake of alcohol, which acts in the body as pure sugar, is high in calories, is void of nutrients, and can cause cravings
- Avoid all artificial sweeteners and caffeinated beverages

For weight loss I recommend eliminating all red meat, dairy products, and wheat. Increase low-fat vegetables and fruits and eat moderate amounts of grains.

PROTEINS (1–2 SERVINGS PER DAY)

2 eggs (3 servings or less per week)	3 oz low-fat cottage cheese	1 c low-fat or nonfat yogurt
3 oz fish (avoid shellfish)	3 oz lean poultry	1 oz spirulina
	2 oz skim mozzarella	⅔ c cooked soybeans
3 oz chicken	4 oz soy protein powder	
3 oz turkey		
3 oz tofu	2 oz skim ricotta	

VEGETABLES (UNLIMITED)

Artichokes	Endives	Pumpkin
Asparagus	Escarole	Radishes
Beets	Garlic	Spinach
Bok choy	Horseradish	Sprouts
Broccoli	Jicama	Swiss chard
Cauliflower	Kale	Turnips
Cabbage	Leeks	Water chestnuts
Celery	Lettuce	Beans, green or yellow
Cucumbers	Onions	

VEGETABLES (3–4 SERVINGS PER WEEK)

Carrots	Yams	Rutabagas
Corn	Okra	Tomatoes
Sweet potatoes	Olives	Squash
Sweet peas	Parsley	Watercress
Potatoes	Peppers	

COMPLEX CARBOHYDRATES: LEGUMES AND GRAINS (3–4 SERVINGS PER DAY)

⅓ c cooked beans

⅓ c cooked brown rice

½ c cooked barley

½ c whole-wheat macaroni

½ c cooked oatmeal

½ c cooked steel-cut oats

½ c cooked amaranth

½ c cooked buckwheat

½ c cooked kasha

½ c cooked spelt

½ c cooked kamut

½ c cooked millet

½ c cooked grits

⅓ c cooked lentils

1 rice cake

1 6-inch corn tortilla

FRUITS (3 SERVINGS PER DAY)

1 small apple

½ c dried fig

½ grapefruit

10 grapes

½ mango

1 small pear

2 plums

1¼ c strawberries

4 medium fresh apricots

¾ c berries

12 cherries

1 peach

¼ of a whole honeydew

¾ of a whole pineapple

2 medium prunes

2 small tangerines

FATS (2 SERVINGS PER DAY)

7 almonds or ½ tsp almond butter

⅓ tsp canola oil

⅓ tsp olive oil

3 olives

⅓ tsp peanut oil

½ tbsp avocado

½ tbsp tahini

1 tsp olive-oil-and-vinegar dressing

½ tsp peanut butter

6 peanuts

FATS (3–4 SERVINGS PER WEEK)

1 tsp mayonnaise

⅓ tsp soybean oil

½ tsp Brazil nuts

⅓ tsp butter

1 tsp cream cheese

⅓ tsp lard

½ tsp sesame oil

½ tsp walnuts

2 tsp bacon bits

½ tbsp cream

½ tbsp light sour cream

⅓ tsp margarine

RECIPES FOR PROTEIN-INTOLERANT DIET

CHILLED PASTA SALAD

Makes 4 servings

>   4 c uncooked whole-wheat macaroni
>   1 tbsp olive oil
>   2 cloves garlic, minced
>   ¹/₂ c chopped broccoli
>   ¹/₂ c chopped cauliflower
>   ¹/₂ c chopped mushrooms
>   ¹/₂ c chopped squash
>   Black pepper to taste
>   6 oz skim ricotta

Cook macaroni as directed on the package; set aside to cool. Heat olive oil and sauté garlic until opaque. Add vegetables and pepper and sauté until tender. While still hot, add vegetables to pasta and crumble in the ricotta cheese. Mix well. Let cool and serve.

ASIAN SALAD

>   ¹/₂ c cabbage
>   ¹/₂ c bok choy
>   ¹/₄ c sprouts
>   ¹/₂ c mushrooms
>   ¹/₄ c water chestnuts
>   1 tsp oil-and-vinegar dressing
>   Black pepper to taste

Chop cabbage, bok choy, sprout, mushrooms, water chesnuts, and toss all ingredients with oil and vinegar, mixing well. Season to taste.

CAULIFLOWER SELDESS

Makes 4 servings

>Cooking spray
>1¹/₂ c raw millet
>2¹/₂ c water
>1 tbsp olive oil
>2 c chopped onion
>1 lb mushrooms, sliced
>Black pepper to taste
>1 tsp dried basil
>1 large cauliflower cut in 1-inch pieces
>3 cloves garlic, minced
>2 tbsp lemon juice
>6 oz grated mozzarella
>Paprika

Spray a 9-by-13-inch pan with nonstick cooking spray. Place the millet and water in a small saucepan. Bring to a boil, cover, and simmer until tender (15 to 20 minutes). Transfer to a large bowl and fluff with a fork.

Heat oil in a large skillet. Add onion, mushrooms, pepper, and basil, and sauté about 5 minutes, until onions soften. Add cauliflower and garlic and sauté about 10 minutes more, until cauliflower is tender. Add lemon juice.

Stir the sautéed vegetables into the millet along with the cheese; mix well. Spread into the prepared pan, dust with paprika, and bake in a 350° oven for 30 minutes.

PERFECT PROTEIN SALAD

Makes 6 servings

>³/₄ c dry soybeans, soaked
>1¹/₂ c cooked white rice
>Black pepper to taste
>¹/₄ c minced fresh dill
>2 tsp low-fat mayonnaise

2 small cloves garlic, minced

$^1/_2$ c finely minced parsley

1 c low-fat cottage cheese

3 scallions, finely minced

1 medium carrot, minced

1 small cucumber, peeled, seeded, and minced

Additional vegetables such as minced onion or celery, fresh alfalfa sprouts, sliced radishes (optional)

Place the soaked soybeans in a medium-sized saucepan and cover with water. Bring to a boil, partially cover, and simmer until tender, about 1–1¼ hours. When the soybeans are still crunchy but tender and the grains are chewy but tender, rinse them in a colander and drain well. Transfer to a bowl. Add all other ingredients and mix well.

BEAN, BARLEY, MUSHROOM, AND EGGPLANT CASSEROLE

Makes 8 servings

2 c barley, cooked

15 oz cooked navy beans

Water

$^3/_4$ tsp dried thyme

$^1/_2$ tsp dried sage

6 cloves garlic, minced

1 tsp black pepper

1 tbsp olive oil

1 c chopped mushrooms

1 c chopped eggplant

$^1/_2$ tsp dried rosemary

6 oz low-fat mozzarella, shredded

Cook 2 cups of barley according to package directions; set aside. Drain beans and reserve liquid; add water to liquid to make 1 cup. Combine cooked barley, beans, thyme, sage, 3 cloves garlic, and pepper; set aside.

Heat oil in a nonstick skillet, add mushrooms and eggplant, remaining garlic, and rosemary; stir well. Sauté 5 minutes. Add bean broth and simmer uncovered for 10 minutes or until all liquid has evaporated.

Coat an 11-by-7-inch baking dish with nonstick spray. Layer half of the bean mixture in the bottom of the dish and top with half of the mozzarella. Add the mushroom and eggplant mixture and cover with the remaining beans and cheese. Bake uncovered at 400° for 25 minutes.

PROTEIN-INTOLERANT DIET — 7-DAY SAMPLE PLAN

MONDAY

BREAKFAST

1 c cooked barley mixed with 4 oz soy protein powder

LUNCH

Tossed salad with cucumbers, beets, mushrooms, and balsamic vinegar
1 small sweet potato, baked, with spray butter and cinnamon
1 small apple

SNACK

6 peanuts

DINNER

4 oz grilled skinless chicken breast in $^1/_2$ whole-wheat pita with $^1/_2$ tbsp
avocado and lettuce, onion, and sprouts

SNACK

1 pear

TUESDAY

BREAKFAST

3 oz low-fat cottage cheese
1 slice whole-wheat bread

LUNCH

> *Chilled Pasta Salad, 1 serving*
> *$^1/_4$ of a whole honeydew*

SNACK

> *12 cherries*

DINNER

> *3 oz tofu, grilled with cooking spray and seasonings*
> *$^2/_3$ c brown rice*
> *Asian Salad*

SNACK

> *10 grapes*

WEDNESDAY

BREAKFAST

> *1 c nonfat yogurt*
> *$^1/_2$ whole-wheat pita, toasted*

LUNCH

> *1 rice cake with 1 tsp peanut butter*
> *$2^1/_2$ medium dates*
> *1 c raw carrots*

SNACK

> *1 c papaya*

DINNER

> *4 oz grilled tuna*
> *$^2/_3$ c cooked lentils with 3 olives*
> *1 c grilled eggplant with oil*

SNACK

$^3/_4$ c pineapple

THURSDAY

BREAKFAST

2 eggs
$^1/_2$ whole-wheat bagel

LUNCH

$^1/_3$ c cooked red beans over $^1/_3$ c brown rice
Salad with kale, lettuce, and sprouts, with $^1/_3$ tsp peanut oil and 1 sliced
orange

SNACK

$1^1/_2$ dried figs

DINNER

4 oz shrimp, boiled or grilled with $^1/_3$ teaspoon canola oil
$^1/_2$ c whole-wheat macaroni
Cauliflower Seldess, 1 c

SNACK

1 peach

FRIDAY

BREAKFAST

$^1/_2$ c cooked oatmeal mixed with 4 oz soy protein powder

LUNCH

Peanut-butter-and-banana sandwich: 2 slices whole-wheat bread,
$^1/_2$ banana, $^1/_2$ tsp peanut butter

SNACK

> *1¹/₂ c strawberries*

DINNER

> *Perfect Protein Salad, 1 serving*

SNACK

> *¹/₂ grapefruit*

SATURDAY

BREAKFAST

> *1 slice whole-wheat bread*
> *2 oz mozzarella melted onto bread*

LUNCH

> *¹/₂ whole-wheat pita, toasted*
> *Tossed salad topped with ¹/₂ mango, balsamic vinegar, and ¹/₃ tsp olive oil*

SNACK

> *2 plums*

DINNER

> *4 oz grilled salmon*
> *²/₃ c cooked black beans with onion*
> *Tossed salad with cucumbers and 1 tsp olive-oil-and-vinegar dressing*

SNACK

> *1 orange*

SUNDAY

BREAKFAST

2 eggs, prepared with cooking spray
$^1/_2$ c cooked grits

LUNCH

$^1/_2$ c cooked millet mixed with $^3/_4$ c berries

SNACK

$^1/_3$ cantaloupe

DINNER

Bean, Barley, Mushroom, and Eggplant Casserole, 1 serving

SNACK

2 small tangerines

12

Conclusion

Recently I sat with over two hundred parents and children at a swimming meet for my daughter, Gabrielle, and her classmates. There I overheard two women sitting directly behind me discussing their specific food intolerances. One woman remarked about the restaurant dinner she and her husband had eaten the night before and how it had caused her a stomach upset that was still with her. She always experienced digestive irritability whenever she ate that particular type of cuisine, and she wondered whether it was caused by the spices, the oil, or the drinks that accompanied the meal. The other woman responded, "Oh, I feel strange after eating almost all foods."

Food allergies are nearly universal, and the bodily aches and pains and the emotional irritability and depression most people experience after eating certain foods are a direct result of their hidden food sensitivities.

Once you have been cleared of food allergies, you will see significant changes in your life: freedom from headaches, indigestion, depression, food cravings, and even arthritis pain and hot flashes. I see this constantly in my clinic, and I teach the self-clearing methods to people every day. As

I mentioned earlier, my daughter, Gabrielle, who is now ten years old, can effectively muscle-test a person and clear food allergies with no special skills other than those I describe in the last two chapters. She can effectively treat herself as well. If a ten-year-old girl can do this, so can you.

Through curing yourself of food allergies I know it is possible to overcome many of the illnesses for which doctors have no solution.

I believe that, for many, BioSET™ is the answer for which they have been searching. For the first time ever, readers now have the BioSET™ technique right at their fingertips. It is my hope that you will enjoy learning these self-healing skills and developing the lifestyle practices that will bring you the health and wellness that you deserve.

Appendix 1

DETOXIFICATION USING HOMEOPATHY

To determine what kind of homeopathic remedies you require, I have put together a questionnaire to help you assess your body's level of toxicity. Once you select your detox remedy, it can be purchased by telephone at (800) 228-1501 or through the Web site at www.wellzymes.com. Also available are audio tapes that provide information on homeopathic detoxification and enzyme formulas.

To complete this questionnaire, answer yes or no to the questions. If you are not sure of an answer, leave that question blank. The recommended homeopathic remedy is listed next to each yes answer. The questionnaire is designed to reveal which of your organs would benefit most from detoxification. Often when you detox one area, the others will improve too. If you answered yes to quite a few questions, I recommend redoing the questionnaire to see which area carries the most stress. It is suggested that you choose no more than three organ formulas at one time.

Do you experience recurrent infections, sinusitis, postnasal drip, or swollen lymph nodes?	Yes (lymph cleanse)	No
Do you experience recurrent respiratory infections, coughs, bronchitis, pneumonia, or asthma?	Yes (lung cleanse)	No
Do you experience bouts of diarrhea, constipation, bloating, or gas?	Yes (colon cleanse)	No

Do you have recurrent yeast infections?	Yes (small intestine cleanse)	No
Do you frequently use antibiotics?	Yes (small intestine cleanse)	No
Do you experience chronic fatigue, recurring infections, or lowered immune response?	Yes (spleen cleanse)	No
Do you experience jaundice, high cholesterol, discomfort in the liver region, or blood disorders?	Yes (liver cleanse)	No
Do you have arthritis, back pain, discomfort when moving, or weather-triggered ailments?	Yes (blood cleanse)	No
Do you have fibromyalgia, rheumatism, carpal tunnel syndrome, or slow recovery after exercise?	Yes (blood cleanse)	No
Do you have skin rashes, dryness or cracking, scaly patches, eczema, or acne or psoriasis?	Yes (skin cleanse)	No
Do you experience edema, gout, or discomfort in the lower back region?	Yes (kidney cleanse)	No
Do you have recurring bladder infections, itching or yeast problems, painful urination, or bed-wetting problems?	Yes (bladder cleanse)	No

CHOOSING THE RIGHT DETOX FORMULA

Remedies that may be beneficial in the healing of various conditions of toxicity can be determined from the preceding list. These remedies are taken in combination with three formulas intended to support specific drainage remedies. These generalized remedies can help to minimize any reactions that might occur from the cleansing effects of detoxification. There are three primary formulas:

- *Drainage*—designed to support detoxification and elimination in various organs and the pancreas.
- *Detox*—designed to reduce toxic load
- *Recharge*—designed to improve energy production, which supports the detoxification process.

This combination of formulas is intended to improve performance, reduce the impact of emotional stress, balance the meridians, enhance detoxification and elimination of a particular organ or system, and relieve symptoms resulting from allergenic reactions.

NOTE: If you experience any discomfort associated with detoxification—such as fatigue, headache, or other symptoms—after beginning the Detox formula, discontinue it, but keep taking the other formulas and increase your intake of water. After one week, restart the Detox formula, but decrease the dose. Two drops will work as well as five drops, but the results may take a little longer.

INSTRUCTIONS FOR TAKING HOMEOPATHIC REMEDIES

Use the dropper in the remedy bottle to place the recommended number of drops onto or under your tongue. Hold the remedy in your mouth at least a few seconds before swallowing to maximize absorption.

Homeopathic remedies are taken on a "clean mouth." That means avoiding food and most beverages half an hour before or after taking the remedy. Also avoid:

- Spicy food or strongly flavored sweets
- Coffee and alcholic beverages
- Smoking
- Use of toothpaste

NOTE: You may also wish to rinse your mouth with bottled or filtered water before taking the remedies.

OTHER TIPS ON HOMEOPATHIC TREATMENT

- Avoid foods that you are sensitive or allergic to, since they may increase symptoms related to toxicity.
- Try to eat only fresh, whole foods and reduce salt, refined sugars, and highly processed foods.
- Chew your food thoroughly to promote complete digestion.
- Drink at least eight eight-ounce glasses of water daily to help flush your system.
- Exercise and deep breathing can help promote the release and elimination of toxins.
- If you experience uncomfortable symptoms related to toxicity, reduce the dosage.

FREQUENTLY ASKED QUESTIONS:

Q: *How should I store my remedies?*

A: The remedies should be kept in a cool, dark place. Make sure the top is screwed on tightly after you use the remedy.

Q: *Will the remedies interfere with my prescription medications?*

A: Homeopathic remedies won't interfere with prescription drugs, but some drugs may block the effects of homeopathic remedies. NOTE: Do not discontinue a prescribed drug without consulting your physician.

THE USE OF ENZYMES

ENZYME QUESTIONNAIRE

This questionnaire, which I created with Dr. Sarah Buchanan, will allow you to evaluate your specific dietary intolerances and then determine the appropriate plant enzyme supplement(s). I recommend taking digestive enzymes immediately before meals or within twenty minutes after. Not only will this prepare the way for the mitigation of your food allergies, but in some cases, it may eliminate some of them immediately. Most importantly, taking enzyme supplements will help you gain optimal health and longevity.

While I do suggest reevaluating yourself periodically, it is not uncommon for a person to require the same enzyme for life. When patients ask me why they need to remain on enzymes permanently, I remind them that if they do not wish to supplement with enzymes, they need to chew each morsel of food at least thirty times so that complete digestion can take place. Anyone who chooses to do this must also remember to eat only organic, wholesome food filled with enzymes and nutrients—which is as important as proper chewing.

I recommend WellZyme products. However, except for enzyme formulas for general digestion, enzyme supplements should not be taken by anyone under sixteen years of age, or by a pregnant or nursing mother, without consulting a BioSET™ practitioner. The exception is the product Digestive Health, which is a multiple enzyme for general digestive support.

QUESTIONNAIRE: WELLZYME CONSUMER NUTRITIONAL ASSESSMENT

Check the box(es) that best describe(s) your symptoms. If you do not know if you have a particular symptom, leave the box blank. The number of the WellZyme product that treats the symptom is given next to the question.

Symptom	WellZyme Product
❑ Weak bones	2
❑ Fatigue, low energy, or extreme stress	3
❑ Seem always to be sick	4
❑ Easily upset stomach	5
❑ Heartburn or pain with eating	5
❑ Problems during menopause	6

❑ Low female sex drive   6

❑ Premenstrual tension or cramping   7

❑ Enlarged prostate   8

❑ Decreased male sex drive or stamina   9

❑ Hay fever or seasonal allergies   11

❑ Develop colds or sinus congestion easily   11

❑ Poor circulation (cold hands or feet)   12

❑ Hemorrhoids or varicose veins   12

❑ Poor eyesight   10

❑ Consistent melancholy mood or feelings of sadness   13

❑ Low motivation to participate in activities   13

❑ Sugar cravings   14

❑ High or low blood sugar   14

❑ Inability to rest adequately   15

❑ Joint weakness or pain/swelling   16

❑ Migraine or severe headaches   17

❑ Problems maintaining mental focus   18

❑ Lung problems   19

❑ Skin (blemishes, scaling, itching)   20

❑ Constipation   21

❑ Dull headache on top of head, psoriasis, fever blisters   22

Do you have a family history of any problems in the following areas?

❑ Heart   12

❑ Poor circulation   12

❑ High blood sugar   14

❑ High cholesterol   12

❑ Eye/vision problems   10

❑ Lung problems   19

❑ Joint problems   16

❑ Weak bones   2

The following are the names of enzyme products from WellZymes, with their corresponding product numbers.

1. Digestive Health (emphasizes sugar and fiber digestion)
2. Bone Health
3. Adrenal Health
4. Immune Health
5. Gastric Ease
6. Mature Woman
7. PMS Comfort
8. Prostate Health
9. Male Vigor
10. Antioxidant
11. Nasal Clear
12. Cardiovascular Health
13. Mood Enhance
14. Blood Sugar Balance
15. Sleep Enhance
16. Joint Health
17. Migra-Min
18. Mental Focus
19. Lung Health
20. Skin, Hair and Nail Health
21. Colon Health
22. Liver Health

THE FOOD ALLERGY KIT

The Food Allergy Kit was originally prepared for Dr. Ellen Cutler's patients for use in home treatment. Given the success of this kit, she wanted to make it available to consumers in conjunction with *The Food Allergy Cure.* The kit contains sample vials of the most prevalent allergens and enables you to test samples of foods and other allergens using the method described in the book.

Remember that even if you don't have the kit, you can use the BioSET™ method at home to clear sensitivities to various foods. Simply have the subject hold a sample of the allergenic food or a sample of the food or beverage in a thin wineglass or glass vial.

The treatment kit is an additional feature that Dr. Cutler has made available to the general public. With the kit, you can also address Level 1 allergies that generally relate to the immune system and the body. This enables you to follow the treatment protocol Dr. Cutler teaches to her patients and considers the most effective approach to clearing food allergies.

The kit contains the Level 1 and 2 allergy vials, as well as a universal blood vial. It is handy and easy to use, with no risk of spoilage. You can also purchase additional food vials, as well as empty vials that will enable you to create your own allergen vials, through Enzymes, Inc.

THE UNIVERSAL BLOOD VIAL

Your blood contains factors produced by your own immune system in response to the foods and substances that trigger your allergies. The blood vial is intended to be used in the BioSET™ method to treat for these immune factors. Using this vial in the treatment sends a message to your immune and nervous systems that desensitize or deprogram the allergen.

To make up your own blood vial, use an empty sterile glass vial, a few drops of distilled water, and a single drop of your blood from a finger stick. You can perform a finger stick with a lancet device available from any pharmacy, or a sterilized needle. Empty vials can be obtained from Enzymes, Inc. Expel a single drop of blood into the empty vial and fill it about half full with distilled water. (You can use this vial instead of the universal blood vial contained in the kit.) Change the blood vial once a month. It does not need to be refrigerated.

Remember that treatment using the blood vial is the very first step of allergy clearing in BioSET™. The blood vial is also used during every subsequent allergy treatment. Be sure that the subject holds his own personal blood vial along with the food or other allergen vial. The use of the blood vial customizes the treatment in response. If the practitioner treats a patient for wheat and uses the individual's blood vial along with the wheat, that individualizes the treatment in a profound way.

Appendix 2

COMMON ALLERGENIC FOODS

The following tables are included in this book so that you will have a complete accounting of common troublesome food items. Many of the foods we eat are mixtures of many ingredients. Because we are not aware of this, we can unknowingly ingest substances to which we are allergic. These tables are meant to inform you about some of the ingredients in many of the packaged and canned foods sitting on grocery store shelves. You can either refrain from eating these foods or, better yet, decide to clear them using the BioSET™ home treatment. Either way, these tables can liberate you from allergic side effects caused by hidden food ingredients.

Foods and Materials Containing Corn or Cornstarch

Adhesives	Beers
Ale	Beets, Harvard
American brandies	Beverages, carbonated
apple	Bleached wheat flours
grape	Bourbon and other whiskies
Aspirin and other tablets	Breads and pastries
Bacon	Cakes
Baking mixes	Candy
Aunt Jemima Pancake Mix	Boxed candies, all grades
Bisquick	Candy bars
Doughnuts	Commercial candies
Baking powders	Carbonated beverages
Batters for frying meat, fish, poultry	Catsup

(continued)

Foods and Materials Containing Corn or Cornstarch (continued)

Cheerios

Cheeses

Chili

Chop suey

Coffee, instant

Confectioner's sugar

Cookies

Corn

    flakes

    flour

    meal

    Mazola corn oil

    parched

    popped

Cough syrups

Cream pies

Cream puffs

Cups, paper

Dates

Deep-fat frying mixtures

Dentifrices

Excipients or diluents in:

    capsules

    suppositories

    tablets

    vitamins

Flour, bleached

Foods, fried

French dressing

Fritos

Frostings

Fruits

Frying fats

Gelatin capsules

Gelatin dessert

Gin

Glucose products

Graham crackers

Grape juice

Gravies

Grits

Gum on envelopes, stickers, stamps, tapes,
    labels

Gums, chewing

Gummed papers

Ham, cured or tenderized

Harvard beets

Holiday-type stickers

Hominy

Ice creams

Ices

Inhalants

    bath powders

    body powders

    cooking fumes from fresh corn

Jams

Jellies

Jell-O

Kremel

Leavening agents

    baking powders

    yeasts

Liquors
  ale
  beer
  gin
  whiskey

Lozenges

Margarine
Meat
  bacon
  bologna
  cooked, with gravies
  frankfurters
  ham, cured or tenderized
  lunch ham
  sausages, cooked
  wieners
Milk, in paper cartons
Monosodium glutamate
Mull-Soy

Nescafe

Ointments

Pablum
Paper containers (only when foods come in
  contact with these containers)
  boxes
  cups
  plates
Pastries
  cakes
  cupcakes
Peanut butters
Peas, canned

Pies, cream
Plastic food wrappers (the inner surfaces
  may be coated with cornstarch)
Powdered sugar
Preserves
Puddings
  blancmange
  custards
  Royal pudding

Salad dressings
Salt
  saltcellars in restaurants
Sandwich spreads
Sauces
  sundaes
  meats
  fish
  vegetables
Seasoned salt
Sherbets
Similac
String beans
  canned
  frozen
Soups
  creamed
  thickened
  vegetable
Soybean milks
  Soya
Starch
  fumes while ironing clothes
Sugar, powdered
Syrups
  commercially prepared glucose syrup
  Karo Syrup

(continued)

Foods and Materials Containing Corn or Cornstarch *(continued)*

Sugars
  Cerelose
  dextrose
  dyno

Talcums
Teas, instant
Toothpaste
Tortillas

Vanillin
Vegetables
  canned

  creamed
  frozen
Vinegar, distilled
Vitamins

Whiskies
  bourbon
  scotch
Wines, American
  dessert
  fortified
  sparkling

Foods Containing Eggs

Baking powder
Batters for frying
Bavarian cream
Boiled dressings
Bouillon
Bread
Breaded foods

Cake flour
Cakes

French toast
Fritters
Frosting

Glazed rolls
Griddle cakes

Hamburger mix
Hollandaise sauce

Ice cream
Ices
Icings

Macaroni
Macaroons
Malted cocoa drinks
  Ovaltine
Marshmallows
Meat jellies
Meat loaf
Meat patties
Meringues

Noodles

Pancake flour
Pancakes
Pastes
Pretzels
Pudding

Salad dressing
Sauces
Sausages
Sherbets
Soufflés
Soups
   consommés
   mock turtle
   noodle

Spaghetti
Spanish creams

Tartar sauce
Timbales

Waffle mixes
Waffles
Wines

Foods Containing Milk

Baking powder biscuits
Bavarian cream
Bisques
Blancmange
Boiled salad dressings
Bread
Butter
Buttermilk
Butter sauces

Cakes
Candies
Cheeses
Chocolate
Chowders
Cocoa drinks, mixtures
Cookies
Cream
Creamed foods
Cream sauces
Curds
Custards

Doughnuts

Eggs, scrambled

Flour mixtures
Foods fried in butter (fish, poultry, beef,
   pork)
Foods prepared au gratin
Fritters

Gravies

Hamburgers
Hard sauces
Hash
Hotcakes

Ice creams

Junket

Malted milk
Margarine
Mashed potatoes
Meat loaf
Milk chocolate

(continued)

Foods Containing Milk (continued)

Omelets	Rarebits
Ovaltine	
	Salad dressings
Pie crust (some)	Sausages, cooked
Prepared mixes	Scalloped dishes
biscuits	Sherbets
cakes	Soda crackers
cookies	Soufflés
doughnuts	Soups
muffins	
pancakes	Whey
pie crust	
waffles	Zwieback

Foods Containing Soybeans

Candies: Soy flours are used in hard candies, fudge, nut candies, custards, and caramels. Soy lecithin is used in candies, particularly chocolate, to prevent drying out and to emulsify the fats.

Cereals

Meats: Pork link sausage and lunch meats can contain soybeans. The allergic individual should buy only pure meat products.

Milk substitutes: Some bakeries use soy milk instead of cow's milk in recipes.

Miscellaneous: Soy products are used in some ice creams and in many soups. Fresh green soy sprouts are served as a vegetable, especially in Chinese dishes. Soybeans are roasted, salted, and used in place of peanuts. They are also used to make soy noodles, macaroons, and spaghetti. Some seasonings contain soy, as do a number of frying fats and shortenings. Margarines and butter substitutes contain the oil and bean products. It is also present in many cookies, crackers, and snacks.

Salad dressings: Many salad dressings and mayonnaises contain soy oil but only list on the label that they contain vegetable oil. When using a particular brand of dressing or mayonnaise, inquire as to the contents.

Note: We are living in an era of expanding uses for soybeans, and the allergy sufferer should anticipate many possible new contacts.

Foods Containing Hidden Sugars

Beverages
  cola drinks
  cordials
  ginger ale
  orange ale
  root beer
  7-Up
  soda pop
  sours
  sweet cider
  whiskey

Cakes and Cookies
  angel food
  applesauce
  banana cake
  brownies
  cheesecake
  chocolate cake
  chocolate cookies
  chocolate éclairs
  coffee cake
  cream puff
  cupcake
  doughnuts
  Fig Newtons
  fruitcake
  gingersnaps
  jelly roll
  macaroons
  nut cookies
  oatmeal cookies
  orange cake
  pound cake
  sponge cake
  strawberry shortcake
  sugar cookies

Candies
  chewing gum
  chocolate cream filling
  chocolate mints
  fudge
  hard candy
  Hershey Bar
  Life Savers
  peanut brittle

Canned Fruits and Juices
  apricots
  apricot syrup
  fruit cocktail
  fruit juice (sweetened)
  fruit syrup
  peaches
  stewed fruits

Dairy Products
  ice cream
  milk shake

Jams, Jellies, and Desserts
  apple butter
  apple cobbler
  custard
  French pastry
  Jell-O
  orange marmalade
  strawberry jelly

Foods Containing Wheat

Beverages
  beer
  cocoa malt
  gin (any drink with grain-neutral spirits)
  malted milk
  Ovaltine
  Postum
  whiskey

Breads
  biscuits
  corn
  crackers
  gluten
  graham
  muffins
  popovers
  pretzels
  rolls
  rye (rye products are not entirely free of
      wheat)
  soy
  wheat

Cereals
  all wheat cereals
  bran flakes
  Corn Flakes
  Cream of Wheat
  Farina
  Grape-Nuts
  other malted cereals
  Puffed Wheat
  Rice Krispies
  Shredded Wheat
  Triscuit
  Wheatena

Flours
  buckwheat
  corn
  gluten
  graham
  lima bean
  patent
  rye
  white
  whole wheat

Pastries and Desserts
  cakes
  candy bars
  chocolate
  cookies
  doughnuts
  pies
  puddings

Wheat Products
  bread
  dumplings
  macaroni
  noodles
  rusks
  spaghetti
  vermicelli
  zwiebacks

Miscellaneous
  bouillon cubes
  chocolate candy
  chocolate (except cocoa and bitter
      chocolate)
  cooked mixed meat dishes
  fats that have been used for frying

foods rolled in flour (including meat)
gravies
griddle cakes
hotcakes
ice cream cones
matzos
mayonnaise
meat
most cooked and prepared meat,
    including sausages, wieners, bologna,

liverwurst, luncheon ham, and
    hamburger
pancake mixes
sauces
synthetic pepper
thickening in ice cream
wheat cakes
wheat germ
waffles
yeasts (some)

Foods Containing Yeast

(The following foods contain yeast as an additive ingredient during preparation, often called leavening)

Breads

Cake and cake mixes
Canned icebox biscuits
Cookies
Crackers

Hamburger buns
Hot dog buns

Meat fried in cracker crumbs
Milk fortified with vitamins from yeast

Pastries
Pretzels

Rolls, homemade or canned

(The following substances contain yeastlike substances because of their nature or the nature of their manufacture or preparation)

Buttermilk

Cheeses of all kinds, including cottage cheese
Citrus fruit juices, frozen or canned (only home-squeezed are yeast-free)

Fermented beverages, including whiskey, wine, brandy, gin, rum, vodka, and root beer

Malted products, including cereals, candy, and malted milk drinks
Mushrooms

Truffles

(continued)

Foods Containing Yeast *(continued)*

Vinegars (apple, pear, grape, and distilled). These may be used alone or in such foods as catsup, mayonnaise, olives, pickles, sauerkraut, condiments, horseradish, French dressing, salad dressing, BBQ sauce, tomato sauce, chili peppers, mince pie and Gerber oatmeal and barley cereal

(The following contain substances that are derived from yeast or have their source in yeast. Read all labels!)

Capsules or tablets containing B vitamins made from yeast
Multiple vitamins
Some enzyme supplements containing brewer's yeast

Appendix 3

Tables of Common Ailments and Food Allergies, Vitamins, and Hormones

DISEASES	RELATED FOOD ALLERGIES
ADHD (attention deficit hyperactivity disorder)	Wheat, dairy, corn products, yeast, chocolate, cinnamon, peanut butter, sulfites, food coloring, MSG, foods that contain salicylates (apples, apricots, blackberries, boysenberries, cantaloupe, cherries, cranberries, currents, dates, guavas, grapes, oranges, pineapples, plums, frozen strawberries, dark red raspberries, gooseberries, tomato paste, radishes, mushrooms, zucchini, peanuts, water chestnuts, and some kinds of crackers), chicories, chili peppers, endive, sweet peppers, almonds, bay leaves, basil, carraway, chili flakes and powder, ginger, mint, nutmeg, cloves, green olives, champagne, white pepper, peppermint, salt, tea bags, herbal teas, vanilla flavoring, wine vinegar, cereals, muffins, biscuits, cakes, coffee, pastries, tobacco, mayonnaise, catsup, gelatin, candies, corned beef, aspirin, and gum
Anorexia	See Weight Problems
Arthritis	Sugar, wheat, citrus, pork, eggs, members of the nightshade family
Asthma (related conditions: chronic bronchitis and chronic sinusitis)	Sulfites used in asthma aerosols and as preservatives (found in dried fruits, prepared potatoes, wine, bottled lemon or lime juice, and shrimp); milk, eggs, peanuts, tree nuts, soy, wheat, fish and shellfish, seeds, soy, citrus fruits, chocolate, coffee, caffeine, spices, animal and vegetable fats, dried beans, yeast, alcohol, baking powder, baking soda, gums, many other grains such as barley and rye, corn and cornstarch
Bulimia	See Weight Problems
Chronic fatigue immune dysfunction syndrome (CFIDS)	Carbohydrates, primarily rice, pasta, grain cereals, and vegetables; wheat, corn, green peas, artichokes, carrots, and most fruits; sugary foods such as fruits, grains, sugared desserts, and chocolate

(continued)

Tables of Common Ailments and Food Allergies, Vitamins, and Hormones (continued)

DISEASES	RELATED FOOD ALLERGIES
Crohn's disease, colitis	Sugars, predominantly lactose, maltose, and glucose; minerals such as zinc and magnesium; the bioflavonoid quercetin; wheat and other gluten-containing grains, including rye, barley, and oats; fiber, such as bran from oats or wheat; artificial sweeteners; dairy, including milk, cheese, and yogurt; vegetables with a high sugar content, such as peas, carrots, and potatoes; nuts; fruits; beans; animal fats and vegetable oils; alcohol, wine, and beer; caffeinated beverages such as cocoa, coffee, and tea; chocolate; carob; yeast; vinegar; food additives; food colorings; modified vegetable starch; sulfites; spices; amino acids such as glutamine
Depression	Vitamin B_{12}, folic acid, vitamin B_1, vitamin B_6, vitamin E, vitamin C; zinc and magnesium; amino acids and phenolics; hormones such as estrogen (found in animal protein, animal liver, alfalfa, soybeans, legumes, anise or fennel, tomato juice, bruised or diseased carrots or potatoes, wheat germ, bran, peanut oil, and licorice); progesterone (found in soy, yams, vegetable oils, beef, and cloves); testosterone (found in turkey); cholesterol (found in animal fats); wheat; milk; sugar; additives such as MSG and aspartame; fermented foods such as pickles; vinegar; caffeine; moldy foods such as yeast and moldy cheeses
Diverticulitis	Grains, legumes, vegetables, fruits
Ear infections	Milk; ice cream; wheat; refined-sugar foods such as candy bars, doughnuts, and muffins; yeast; corn; soy; peanuts; eggs; oranges; tomatoes; chicken
Eczema	Milk, eggs, peanuts, sugars, soy, wheat, citrus, fruit juices, food additives, sulfites, artificial colors, gums, tomatoes, meat and fish products, pickles, relishes, vanilla, fats, chocolate
Gastritis	Fatty foods, alcohol, chocolate, spicy foods, peppermint, citrus, tomatoes, coffee, peppers, calcium supplements
Headaches and migraines	All alcoholic beverages, especially red wine, champagne, beer, vodka, port; black tea and green tea with caffeine; coffee; chocolate; meats such as sausage, bologna, salami, pepperoni, hot dogs, ham, pork, Spam, organ meats, game meats, and meat

DISEASES	RELATED FOOD ALLERGIES
	tenderizers; fish such as sardines and herring; salt; dried fruits; preservatives; artificial sweeteners; corn; milk; yogurt; nuts, especially cashews; soy products, such as soy sauce, tofu, tempeh, and tamari; wheat; spices; food additives, including nitrates; food preservatives, such as benzoic acid and tartrazine; smoked cured meat; overripe fruits; apples; citrus; certain types of fruit juices and fruit chemicals; sugars; members of the nightshade family, such as potatoes, tomatoes, turnips, and peppers; sourdough bread; doughnuts; yeast extracts; overuse of analgesic medications such as aspirin and Tylenol
Hives	Peanuts, eggs, shellfish, tomatoes, chocolate, nuts, spices, milk, food additives, artificial sugars, prescription or over-the-counter drugs
Infertility (male and female)	Yeast, dairy products, grains, fruits, parsley, dill, fennel, legumes, soybeans, tomatoes, wheat, peanuts, licorice, high-retinol foods such as carrots, green vegetables, yellow vegetables, broccoli, chard, spinach, egg yolk, liver, kidney, raw whole peaches, halibut, salmon, cream cheese, butter, apricots, mackerel, crab, oysters, swordfish, kale, sweet potatoes, melons, papaya, grapefruit, fish liver oils
Irritable bowel syndrome	Refined sugar; high-fiber foods such as brown rice; oats; high-fiber vegetables such as beans, peas, and lentils; raw fruits, especially citrus, apples, grapes, raisins, cantaloupe, and bananas; fatty foods such as meats, poultry, fish, potato chips, french fries, onion rings, and all vegetable and animal oils; dairy products, more specifically the sugar lactose; wheat; coffee; tea
Menopausal symptoms	Vitamins such as vitamin B_6, B_5, PABA, vitamin C, and bioflavonoids; minerals such as calcium and magnesium; hormones such as estrogen and progesterone; foods such as soybeans, flaxseed, vegetables, parsley, dill, fennel, dairy products, rice, wheat, salt, seaweed, beef, pork, chicken, salmon, flounder, tuna, crab, shrimp, barley, rice, peanuts, sesame, dried apricots, avocadoes, dates, pecans, almonds, cashews, Brazil nuts, corn, sunflower seeds, rapeseed, alfalfa, lettuce,

(continued)

Tables of Common Ailments and Food Allergies, Vitamins, and Hormones
(continued)

DISEASES	RELATED FOOD ALLERGIES
	sweet potatoes, egg yolk, butter, cream, olive oil, wheat germ
Osteoporosis	Calcium and magnesium
PMS—premenstrual syndrome	Hormones such as estrogen and progesterone; minerals such as calcium and magnesium; vitamins such as vitamin E and B vitamins; foods such as animal fats, alcohol, sugars, caffeine, pesticides, meats, dairy products
Weight problems (including anorexia and bulimia)	All carbohydrates; sugars; all grains, especially wheat, barley, and rye; all animal and vegetable fats; food additives; food coloring; alcoholic beverages, including red wine, white wine, and beer; yeast; vegetables such as carrots, peas, potatoes, yams, and sweet potatoes; chocolate; dairy products

FOOD	ASSOCIATED PHYSICAL ILLNESS WHEN ALLERGIC
Alcoholic beverages	Weakness in bones, insomnia, arthritis, headaches, depression, kidney stones, candida infections, bloating, asthma
Animal fats	Increased menopausal and premenstrual symptoms, premenstrual headaches, menstrual cramping, excess weight gain, arthritic pain, constipation
Barley, oats, and rye	Symptoms of the digestive system (bloating and gas) and skin (dry skin and eczema)
Breast milk	In babies: upset stomach, poor disposition, poor eating, poor sleeping habits
Caffeine, chocolate, and coffee	Migraines, arthritis pain, heartburn, breast tenderness, endometriosis, asthma, coughing, sinus congestion
Carrots	Asthma, migraines, eczema
Corn	Migraines, arthritis, digestive problems
Cucumbers	Chronic fatigue, nasal congestion, arthritis, sugar craving, migraines

FOOD	ASSOCIATED PHYSICAL ILLNESS WHEN ALLERGIC
Dairy products—milk, yogurt, and cheese	Excess mucus production, arthritis, digestive problems
All dried beans and legumes (garbanzo, kidney, pinto, navy, soy, black, red, lima, mung, fava)	Digestive problems, headaches, migraines
Eggs	Excess mucus production, arthritis, headaches
Fish and seafood	Eczema, asthma, migraines, digestive problems, sinus congestion, gout, arthritis
Food coloring	Severe constriction of the air passageways, coughing, runny nose, fever, hives, migraines, hyperactivity, insomnia, depression, attention deficit hyperactivity disorder
Fruits	Excess mucus production, asthma attacks
Garlic	Asthma, indigestion, bloating, headaches
MSG	Migraines, visual disturbances, erratic behavior, asthma, hives, severe anaphylactic reactions
Nightshades (eggplants, potatoes, tomatoes, and peppers)	Arthritis, joint pain, migraines, digestive problems
Peanuts, cashews, pecans, walnuts	Excess mucus production, asthmatic attacks, anaphylactic shock, migraines, digestive problems
Peppers	Arthritis, depression, impotence, sinus congestion, headaches, digestive problems
Pesticides	Headaches, arthritis, breast pain, skin reactions, depression, hyperactivity, irritability
Potatoes	Arthritis, chronic fatigue, headaches and migraines, weight problems (including anorexia and bulimia)
Salicylates	Asthma, digestive problems, nasal congestion, sleep problems, tongue lesions, hyperactivity
Salt	Water retention, high blood pressure, coughs, and headaches; correlated with asthma deaths in men and children and increased bronchial activity in men (but not in women)

(continued)

Tables of Common Ailments and Food Allergies, Vitamins, and Hormones (continued)

FOOD	ASSOCIATED PHYSICAL ILLNESS WHEN ALLERGIC
Soy products	Chronic ear infections, eczema, chronic upper respiratory infections, severe bloating, gas, asthma
Sugars	Chronic immune deficiencies, mucus in the throat and respiratory system, asthma, chronic coughs, malabsorption of vitamins and minerals, indigestion, mood swings, weight problems, arthritis pain, muscle and joint pain, depression, food cravings; in children, attention problems, chronic ear infections, sore throats, sinus congestion
Sulfites	Asthma
Vegetable oils	Increased menopausal and premenstrual symptoms, menstrual cramping, excess weight gain, arthritic pain, constipation
Water	Excess mucus, coughing, asthma, severe bloating, eczema, hives
Wheat	Fatigue, eczema, arthritis, digestive problems, colitis, food cravings, brain fog
Yams	Migraine, headache, obesity, canker sores, depression, asthma, arthritis, attention deficit hyperactivity disorder, eczema, digestive problems, sugar craving

HORMONE	ALLERGY SYMPTOM	FOODS CONTAINING HORMONE
Cholesterol	Asthma, breast pain, chest pain, elevated cholesterol, gallbladder problems, gallstones, headache, heart problems, slow healing, scalp tightness	Animal fats
Estrogen	Depression, dizziness, emotional instability, fibrocystic breast disease, fuzzy head, generalized itching, hormonal	Animal protein, alfalfa, soybeans, legumes, anise or fennel, tomato juice, bruised or diseased carrots or pota-

HORMONE	ALLERGY SYMPTOM	FOODS CONTAINING HORMONE
	imbalance, hot flashes, infertility, irregular periods, manic-depressive illness, nervousness, premenstrual syndrome, postpartum psychosis, seizures, shakiness, sleepiness, spontaneous abortion, infertility, throbbing headache, vaginal burning, painful intercourse, thinning of vaginal mucosa	toes, wheat germ, bran, peanut oil, licorice
Progesterone	Aching legs, backache, burning in the back of the head, pressure in the chest, depression, dysmenorrhea, fibrocystic breast disease, fuzzy or foggy head, gas, head pressure, headache, heart problems, hot flashes, itching scalp and hands, menstrual cramps, nausea, premenstrual syndrome, nervousness, sleep disorders, weepiness	Soy, yams, vegetable oils, beef, cloves
Testosterone	Acne, impotence, hirsutism, low sex drive, overaggressiveness in males, sleep problems	Turkey

Tables of Common Ailments and Food Allergies, Vitamins, and Hormones

VITAMIN OR MINERAL	FUNCTION IN BODY	SYMPTOMS OF ALLERGY/ DEFICIENCY	FOUND IN THESE ALLERGENIC FOODS
Vitamin A/beta-carotene	Immunostimulant; antioxidant; healthy mucous membranes; prevents colds, acne, skin disorders, flu, respiratory infections. Heals ulcers and wounds; promotes growth of bones, teeth, good vision. Common asthma treatment.	Skin tags, warts, blemishes, acne, rashes, hair loss, premature aging; bronchial, lung, and respiratory problems; lowered immunity; infertility; joint pain; vomiting; GI problems	Papayas, peaches, other yellow fruit, asparagus, beets, broccoli, carrots, Swiss chard, kale, turnip greens, watercress, parsley, red peppers, sweet potatoes, squash, yellow squash, other yellow vegetables, pumpkin, corn, spirulina, milk, butter, other dairy products, egg yolk, fish, fish liver oil
B vitamins (general)—these vitamins are synergistic and work better when taken together	Essential for emotional, physical, and psychological well-being; maintain a healthy nervous system; aid in the digestion of fats, carbohydrates, and protein	Skin disorders, respiratory problems, colds, poor memory, hair loss, anemia, severe depression, cloudy thinking, exhaustion, mood swings, nervousness, chronic fatigue, eczema, arthritis, stress	Found in all foods except tapioca, Jell-O, and Cool Whip
B$_1$/thiamin	Aids in the metabolic utilization of carbohydrates; stabilizes the appetite; promotes growth &	Loss of appetite and weight, feelings of weakness and tiredness, paralysis, nervousness,	Bread, cereals, pasta, and rice; meat, especially pork, poultry, and fish; fruits;

VITAMIN OR MINERAL	FUNCTION IN BODY	SYMPTOMS OF ALLERGY/ DEFICIENCY	FOUND IN THESE ALLERGENIC FOODS
	good muscle tone; inhibits pain; assists in the normal functioning of the nervous system, muscles, and heart	irritability, insomnia, unfamiliar aches and pains, depression, heart difficulties, constipation and gastrointestinal problems, beriberi	vegetables; sunflower seeds
B_2/riboflavin	Metabolizes carbohydrates, fats, and protein; maintains cell respiration, vision, healthy nails and hair; makes antibodies and red blood cells	Sluggishness; itching, burning, or bloodshot eyes; sores or cracks in and around the mouth and lips; purplish or inflamed tongue and mouth; dermatitis; oily skin; slowed growth; trembling; digestive and respiratory problems	Breads, cereals, and other grain products, milk and milk products, meat, poultry, fish
B_3/niacin	Improves circulation, reduces "bad" cholesterol, raises "good" cholesterol, maintains the nervous system, healthy skin, tongue, and digestion, tissue respiration, and fat synthesis. Aids in metabolizing protein, sugar and fat. Helps to reduce high	Gastrointestinal disturbance, loss of appetite, indigestion, bad breath, canker sores, skin disorders or rashes, muscular weakness, fatigue, insomnia, vague aches and pains, headaches, nervousness, memory loss, irritability or depression, res-	Meat, poultry, fish (especially tuna), bread, cereals, wheat bran, mushrooms, asparagus, peanuts

(continued)

Tables of Common Ailments and Food Allergies, Vitamins, and Hormones (continued)

VITAMIN OR MINERAL	FUNCTION IN BODY	SYMPTOMS OF ALLERGY/ DEFICIENCY	FOUND IN THESE ALLERGENIC FOODS
	blood pressure, metabolizes sex hormones, activates histamines, and prevents pellagra.	piratory problems, pellagra	
B_5/pantothenic acid	Aids in detoxification, digestion of fats, carbohydrates, and proteins. Maintains the nervous system and the immune system and healthy skin. Supports the adrenal glands to produce cortisol in times of stress; fights infection by building antibodies; stimulates growth. Helps build cells and utilize vitamins.	Asthma, muscle cramping, painful and burning feet, skin abnormalities, retarded growth, dizzy spells, weakness, depression, decreased resistance to infection, restlessness, digestive disturbances, stomach stress, vomiting	Rice, molasses, yeast, milk, whole grains, cereals, beef and pork liver, beef, chicken, salmon, mackerel, sardines, lobsters, clams, crabs, mushrooms, avocadoes, watermelon, pineapples, soy, lentils, bean sprouts, peanuts
B_6/pyridoxine, pyridoxal-5-phosphate	Necessary for synthesis and breakdown of DNA, RNA, and amino acids. Required for normal functioning of the brain. Aids in metabolism of fat and carbohydrates, the formation of	Carpal tunnel syndrome, joint pain, homocystinuria, sensitivity to bright light, sensitivity to MSG, burning or tingling in the extremities, inability to recall dreams, imbalances of the	Meat, poultry, fish, fruits, vegetables, grain products, ready-to-eat and instant cereals

VITAMIN OR MINERAL	FUNCTION IN BODY	SYMPTOMS OF ALLERGY/ DEFICIENCY	FOUND IN THESE ALLERGENIC FOODS
	antibodies, and lessening of discomfort during the menstrual period. Aids hemoglobin in its function; promotes healthy skin; reduces muscle spasms, leg cramps, and stiffness of the hands; helps to prevent nausea and promotes the balance of sodium and phosphorus in the body.	liver, dermatitis, loss of muscular control, muscle weakness, arm and leg cramps, fatigue, nervousness, irritability, insomnia, slow learning, water retention, anemia, mouth disorders, hair loss	
B_{12}	Builds red blood cells and genetic material; metabolizes carbohydrates, fats, and proteins; increases energy; maintains nervous system and muscles; promotes cell longevity, memory, appetite, digestive system, immune system. Aids in absorption of iron and calcium, prevents inflammation, assists in folate metabolism and	Pernicious anemia, degeneration of spinal cord and nerves, poor appetite, stunted growth (in children), nervousness, depression, lack of balance, neuritis, brain damage, paleness and sallow complexion, shiny or sore red tongue, weakness and fatigue progressing to paralysis, numbness or tingling in hands and feet,	Meat, eggs, milk products, edible seaweeds, certain mushrooms, sourdough bread, tofu, tempeh, miso, barley malt syrup, parsley, beer, cider, wine, port, margarine, fortified nutritional yeast, fortified breakfast cereals, soy milk and other soy products, clams, oysters, organ meats

(continued)

Tables of Common Ailments and Food Allergies, Vitamins, and Hormones
(continued)

VITAMIN OR MINERAL	FUNCTION IN BODY	SYMPTOMS OF ALLERGY/ DEFICIENCY	FOUND IN THESE ALLERGENIC FOODS
	DNA synthesis, insulates nerve fibers, converts fat to lean muscle and iron to hemoglobin. Helps normalize hormones, improves short-term memory in the elderly. An anti-aging nutrient.	gradual deterioration of motor coordination, moodiness, poor memory, confusion, delirium, delusion, hallucinations and psychotic states	
Folic acid	Helps in formation of red blood cells and genetic material, in growth and reproduction of body cells, in amino acid conversion, in breakdown and assimilation of protein, and in the formation of nucleonic acid. Stimulates appetite, maintains healthy intestinal tract, may reverse certain types of anemia, reduces risk of cervical dysplasia, lowers risk for heart attack. During pregnancy, protects fetus against birth anom-	Megaloblastic anemia, GI disorders, prematurely gray hair, pale tongue, vitamin B_{12} deficiency	Citrus fruits, tomatoes, green leafy vegetables, grain products, organ meats

VITAMIN OR MINERAL	FUNCTION IN BODY	SYMPTOMS OF ALLERGY/ DEFICIENCY	FOUND IN THESE ALLERGENIC FOODS
	alies and reduces risk of premature birth.		
Biotin	Strengthens immune system. Aids in cell growth; fatty acid production and synthesis; formation of DNA and RNA; and utilization of protein, folic acid, pantothenic acid and vitamin B_{12}. Produces healthy hair.	Inability to properly absorb any B vitamins, drowsiness, extreme exhaustion, depression, loss of appetite, muscle pain, gray skin color	Brewer's yeast, rice, soy, liver, kidneys, milk, molasses, nuts, fruits, beef, egg yolk
Inositol	Necessary for growth of muscle cells and formation of lecithin. Aids in fat breakdown, reduces cholesterol, helps prevent thinning hair. Calming, antioxidant.	Hair loss, eczema, constipation, migraines, high blood cholesterol	Citrus fruits, grain cereal, grains, meats, organ meats, wheat germ, barley, oats, yeast, molasses, chicken, salmon, peanuts, apple, raisins, strawberries
Choline	Controls fat and cholesterol buildup, prevents fat from accumulating in the liver, and facilitates movement of fats in cells and throughout the bloodstream. Helps regulate kidneys, liver, and gall-	Cirrhosis and fatty degeneration of liver, hardening of arteries, heart problems, high blood pressure, hemorrhaging kidneys	Brewer's yeast, wheat germ, egg yolk, liver, green leafy vegetables, legumes, peas, beans, heart, lecithin

(continued)

Tables of Common Ailments and Food Allergies, Vitamins, and Hormones *(continued)*

VITAMIN OR MINERAL	FUNCTION IN BODY	SYMPTOMS OF ALLERGY/ DEFICIENCY	FOUND IN THESE ALLERGENIC FOODS
	bladder. Maintains myelin sheaths, facilitates nerve transmission, improves memory, and supports brain chemistry.		
PABA/para-aminobenzoic acid	Antioxidant, membrane stabilizer, prevents red blood cells and lysosomal membranes from bursting, helps bacteria produce folic acid, aids in formation of red blood cells and assimilation of pantothenic acid. Produces healthy skin and skin pigmentation, helps return gray hair to its natural color, screens skin from sun exposure.	Extreme fatigue, irritability, depression, nervousness, eczema, constipation, digestive disorders, headaches, premature graying of hair	Brewer's yeast, liver, heart, kidneys, wheat germ, yogurt, leafy green vegetables, molasses
Vitamin C	Essential for action of folic acid in manufacture of blood cells, normal function of the endocrine glands, synthesis of colla-	Scurvy, tiredness, lethargy, exhaustion, chronic sore throat, eczema, colds and flu	Rose hips, citrus fruits, black currants, apples, strawberries, guavas, cherries, potatoes, cabbage, broccoli, tomatoes, turnip

VITAMIN OR MINERAL	FUNCTION IN BODY	SYMPTOMS OF ALLERGY/ DEFICIENCY	FOUND IN THESE ALLERGENIC FOODS
	gen, synthesis of adrenal cortical hormones, and prevention of cholesterol buildup.		greens, green bell peppers, leafy green vegetables, cauliflower, sweet potatoes
Vitamin E	A fat-soluble antioxidant that protects cells from free radical damage and neutralizes the damaging effects of ozone.	Hypertension, breast tenderness, cysts and congestion, hot flashes, menopause symptoms, muscular dystrophy, varicosities, acne, poor healing, toxicity, oxidative stress, generalized edema, faulty absorption of fat and fat-soluble vitamins	Wheat germ or wheat germ oil, vegetable oils, soybeans or soybean oil, green vegetables, flours, grains, eggs, raw nuts, sprouted seeds, fish
Vitamin F/fatty acids (general)	Needed for the absorption of vitamins A, D, K, and beta-carotene. Helps slow release of sugar into bloodstream.	Integrity of cell membranes weakened, nervous system problems, weak immune system, hypoglycemia, diabetes, skin allergies	Vegetable oils, wheat germ oil, linseed oil, sunflower oil, safflower oil, soybean oil, peanuts or other nuts, peanut oil, flaxseed or flaxseed oil, evening primrose oil, breast milk
Omega-6 fatty acids	Fights inflammation.	Arthritis, dry skin, eczema, high cholesterol, retarded growth, hormone problems	All vegetable oils, most grains, beans

(continued)

Tables of Common Ailments and Food Allergies, Vitamins, and Hormones
(continued)

VITAMIN OR MINERAL	FUNCTION IN BODY	SYMPTOMS OF ALLERGY/ DEFICIENCY	FOUND IN THESE ALLERGENIC FOODS
Omega-3 fatty acids	Turn into prostaglandins E1 and E3 and reduce inflammation.	Arthritis, hormone problems, premature aging of skin and hair, impotence, high blood pressure, depressed immune system, poor nail growth, low strength	Flaxseed, flaxseed oil, fresh walnuts, walnut oil, pumpkin seeds, soybean oil, canola oil
Calcium	Essential for maintenance of body's bones and nervous system.	Joint pain or aches, osteoporosis, menstrual leg cramps, tetany, headache, hyperactivity, restlessness, abdominal pain, insomnia, skin problems, nervousness, canker sores, herpes, hyperactivity, obesity, arthritis pain, inability to relax	Milk, dairy products, root and green vegetables, sesame seeds, oats, beans, almonds, walnuts, peanuts, sunflower seeds, sardines, salmon
Iron	Aids in growth, promotes resistance to disease, and prevents fatigue.	Anemia, chronic iron deficiency problems, backaches, headaches, dizziness, menstrual problems, fatigue	Apricots, peaches, bananas, prunes, raisins, blackstrap molasses, brewer's yeast, whole grains, cereals, turnip greens, spinach, beets, beet tops, alfalfa, asparagus, kelp, sunflower seeds, walnuts,

VITAMIN OR MINERAL	FUNCTION IN BODY	SYMPTOMS OF ALLERGY/ DEFICIENCY	FOUND IN THESE ALLERGENIC FOODS
Zinc	Key nutrient in skin health.	Eczema and acne	sesame seeds, beans, egg yolk, liver, red meat, oysters, clams Green leafy vegetables, pork, beef, lamb, fish, brown rice, eggs, milk, brewer's yeast, mushrooms, onions, peas, beans, seeds, wheat bran, wheat germ, herring, oysters, mustard

Bibliography

ALLERGY INFORMATION

The research on allergies is extensive. Currently the Medline database of the National Library of Medicine, National Institutes of Health (NIH), contains hundreds of thousands of entries on allergies. Terms used to classify the research on allergies include:

- *Allergy:* "Hypersensitivity caused by exposure to a particular allergen (antigen) resulting in a marked increase in reactivity... upon subsequent exposure sometimes resulting in harmful immunologic consequences."[1] (Medline includes 165,114 abstract summaries under the general term "allergy.")
- *Hypersensitivity:* "Altered reactivity to an antigen, which can result in pathologic reactions upon subsequent exposure to that particular antigen."[2] (Medline entries— 169,096)
- *Hypersensitivity, Delayed:* "An increased reactivity to specific antigens mediated not by antibodies but by cells."[3] (Medline entries— 19,714)
- *Hypersensitivity, Immediate:* "Hypersensitivity reactions which occur within minutes of exposure to challenging antigen due to the release of histamine which follows the antigen-antibody reaction and causes smooth muscle contraction and increased vascular permeability."[4] (Medline entries— 7,159)
- *Immune Complex Diseases:* "A group of diseases mediated by the deposition of large soluble complexes of antigen and antibody with resultant damage to tissue...[linked to]

1. *Stedman's Medical Dictionary,* 26th ed. Philadelphia, PA: Lippincott, Williams & Wilkins, 1995.
2. PubMed, National Library of Medicine, National Institutes of Health. www.ncbi.nlm.nih.gov/PubMed/. Accessed 3/02.
3. Ibid.
4. Ibid.
5. Ibid.

systemic immunologic diseases including [certain forms of kidney disease] and systemic lupus."[5] (Medline entries—7,159)

The following ten abstracts provide a sense of the breadth of the topic.

Geha, R. S., and others. "Multicenter, double-blind, placebo-controlled, multiple-challenge evaluation of reported reactions to monosodium glutamate." *Journal of Allergy and Clinical Immunology.* 2000; vol. 106: 973–80.

Greenberger, P. A., and M. J. Flais. "Bee pollen–induced anaphylactic reaction in an unknowingly sensitized subject." *Annals of Allergy, Asthma, and Immunology.* 2001; vol. 86: 239–42.

Kalliomaki, M., and others. "Probiotics in primary prevention of atopic disease." *Lancet.* 2001; vol. 357: 1076–79.

Lee, M. J. "Parasites, yeast, and bacteria in health and disease." *Journal of Advancement in Medicine.* Summer 1995; vol. 8, no. 2: 121 and l27–28.

Majamaa, H., and E. Isolauri. "Probiotics: a novel approach in the management of food allergy." *Journal of Allergy and Clinical Immunology.* 1997; vol. 99: 179–85.

Sicherer, S. H. "Diagnosis and management of childhood food allergy." *Current Problems in Pediatrics.* 2001; vol. 31: 35–62.

Skolnick, H. S., and others. "The natural history of peanut allergy." *Journal of Allergy and Clinical Immunology.* 2001; vol. 107: 367–74.

Taylor, S., and S. L. Hefle. "Will genetically modified foods be allergenic?" *Journal of Allergy and Clinical Immunology.* 2001; vol. 107: 765–71.

Vadas, P., and others. "Detection of peanut allergens in breast milk of lactating women." *Journal of the American Medical Association.* 2001; vol. 285: 1746–48.

Vander Leek, T. K., and others. "The natural history of peanut allergy in young children and its association with serum peanut-specific IgE." *Journal of Pediatrics.* 2000; vol. 137: 749–55.

MUSCLE TESTING— APPLIED KINESIOLOGY

The 8th Annual Congress of the Japan Bi-Digital O-Ring Test Medical Society. Tokyo, Japan. July 19–20, 1998. Abstracts in *Acupuncture Electrotherapy Research.* 1998; vol. 23: 207–31.

The 9th Annual Congress of the Japan Bi-Digital O-Ring Test Medical Society. Tokyo, Japan. July 24–25, 1999. Abstracts in *Acupuncture Electrotherapy Research.* 1999; vol. 24: 203–33.

Kail, K. "Clinical outcomes of a diagnostic and treatment protocol in allergy/sensitivity patients." *Alternative Medicine Review.* 2001; vol. 6: 188–202. [This reference focuses on electrodermal screening, a technique used by BioSET™ practitioners in allergy testing.]

Monti, D. A., and others. "Muscle test comparisons of congruent and incongruent self-referential statements." *Perceptual Motor Skills.* Jun 1999; vol. 88, no. 3 pt. 1: 1019–28.

Ogata, H., T. Matsumoto, and H. Tsukahara. "Changes in the electrical skin resistance on meridians during gastric surgery under general anesthesia." *American Journal of Chinese Medicine.* 1983; vol. 11: 123–29.

Omura, Y. "New simple early diagnostic methods using Omura's 'Bi-Digital O-Ring Dysfunction Localization Method' and acupuncture organ representation points, and their applications to the 'drug and food compatibility test.'" *Acupuncture Electrotherapy Research.* 1981; vol. 6, no. 4: 239–54.

Schmitt, W. H., Jr., and G. Leisman. "Correlation of applied kinesiology muscle testing findings with serum immunoglobulin levels for food allergies." *International Journal of Neuroscience.* Dec 1998; vol. 96, no. 3–4: 237–44.

ACUPRESSURE AND ACUPOINTS

The BioSET™ technique used to reprogram the nervous and immune systems is a form of gentle acupressure, applied first to various acupoints on the back, then to the arms and legs. The specific points on the back extend the length of the spine, located on either side of and about an inch from the vertebrae. These points occur on an important meridian recognized in traditional Chinese medicine as the bladder meridian. The points are also referred to as association points. Acupuncturists have noted that these points exert a particularly beneficial influence on the body, and research has found that they affect and improve symptoms associated with other meridians. Consequently, they appear to have a major influence on the energetic system of the entire body.

Debreceni, L. "On the possible specific role of acupuncture loci [particularly the associ-ation points] in therapeutics." *Complementary Medicine East and West.* Summer 1977; vol. 5, no. 2: 177–79.

Jiang, H., and Z. Yang. "Influence of finger pressing massage on cAMP and cGMP [nucleotides] in the cerebrospinal fluid in prolapsed intervertebral disc." [Article in Chinese.] *Zhong Xi Yi Jie He Za Zhi.* Jan 1990; vol. 10, no. 1: 27–29.

Kotani, N., and others. "Preoperative intradermal acupuncture [of association points] reduces postoperative pain, nausea and vomiting, analgesic requirement, and sympathoadrenal responses." *Anesthesiology.* 2001; vol. 95: 349–56.

Sun, Y. "External approach to the treatment of pediatric asthma." *Journal of Traditional Chinese Medicine.* 1995; vol. 15: 290–91.

———. "Fourteen cases of child bronchial asthma treated by auricular plaster and meridian instrument." *Journal of Traditional Chinese Medicine.* 1998; vol. 18: 202–4.

Zhang, Y. "Observation of curative effects of Huatuojiaji [bladder meridian—association points] in the treatment of 300 cases of apoplexy (stroke)." *Journal of Traditional Chinese Medicine.* Jun 1996; vol. 16, no. 2: 117–20.

NUTRITION

Bland, J. S. *Nutritional Improvement of Health Outcomes: The Inflammatory Disorders.* Gig Harbor, WA: Institute for Functional Medicine, 1997.

Bland, J. S., and others. *Clinical Nutrition: A Functional Approach.* Gig Harbor, WA: Institute for Functional Medicine, 1999.

Great Smokies Diagnostic Laboratory (GSDL). *Comprehensive Digestive Stool Analysis Application Guide.* Asheville, NC: GSDL, 1998.

Kannel, W. B. "The Framingham Study." *Journal of Atherosclerosis and Thrombosis.* 2000; vol. 6, no. 2: 60–66.

Kant, A. K., and others. "A prospective study of diet quality and mortality in women." *Journal of the American Medical Association.* 2000; vol. 283: 2109–15.

Lincinio, P., and others. "A molecular mechanism for stress-induced alterations in susceptibility to disease." *Lancet.* 1995; vol. 346: 104–6.

PDR Physicians' Desk Reference for Nonprescription Drugs and Dietary Supplements. Montvale: Medical Economics Data, 2000.

Shils, M., and others, eds. *Modern Nutrition in Health and Disease,* 9th ed. Baltimore: Lippincott, Williams & Wilkins, 1999.

Werbach, M. R. *Nutritional Influences on Illness: A Sourcebook of Clinical Research,* 2nd ed. Tarzana, CA: Third Line Press, Inc., 1996.

Williams, R. J. *Biochemical Individuality: the Basis for the Genetotropic Concept.* New York: Keats/NTC Contemporary, Inc., 1998.

DETOXIFICATION

BOOKS AND WEB SITES

Bennett, P., S. Faye, S. Barrie, and J. Miller, eds. *7-Day Detox Miracle.* Rocklin, CA: Prima Publishing, 2001.

Bland, J., and S. H. Benum. *The 20-Day Rejuvenation Diet Program.* New York: Keats/NTC Contemporary, Inc., 1999.

Krohn, J., F. A. Taylor, and J. Posser. *Natural Detoxification.* Vancouver, Canada: Harley & Marks Publishers Inc., 1996.

Metagenics, Inc. Information on detoxification: www.metagenics.com.

Murray, M. T., and J. Pizzorno. *The Encyclopedia of Natural Medicine.* Rocklin, CA: Prima Publishing, 1998.

Pizzorno, J. *Total Wellness.* Rocklin, CA: Prima Publishing, 1998.

Scott-Moncrieff, C. *Detox: Cleanse and Recharge Your Mind, Body and Soul.* New York: Collins & Brown, 2001.

LITERATURE REVIEW—EXAMPLE: THE ROLE OF TOXICITY IN KIDNEY DISORDERS

The interplay between toxicity and immune response may be greater than is generally appreciated. One way to explore the subject of toxicity is by focusing on a particular health issue. For example, a Medline search on "toxin and connective tissue" yielded 1,542 citations. A search on the role of toxicity in kidney disorders, using the keywords "toxin and kidney," yielded 6,035 citations. The first fifty research articles linked both environmental toxins and infectious processes to kidney disorders, including:

- External toxins such as heavy metals, mercury, and Chinese herbs
- Infectious agents, including campylobacter, candida, clostridium, E. coli, mold (aflatoxins), mycotoxins, and Shiga toxin (most pathogens are known to produce toxins)
- Infectious processes, including sepsis, and endotoxins produced by the body

ENZYME THERAPY

Balch, J. F. and P. A. Balch. *Prescription for Nutritional Healing.* 2nd ed. Garden City Park, NY: Avery Publishing Group, Inc., 1997.

Cichoke, A. J. *The Complete Book of Enzyme Therapy.* Garden City Park, NY: Avery Publishing Group Inc., 1999.

Holford, Ellen. *The Optimum Nutrition Bible.* Freedom, CA: Crossing Press, 1999, 105–9.

Howell, E. *Enzyme Nutrition: The Food Enzyme Concept.* Wayne, NJ: Avery Publishing Group, Inc., 1985.

———. *Food Enzymes for Health and Longevity.* Woodstock Valley, CT: Omangod Press, 1980.

Lopez, D. A., R. M. Williams, K. Miehlke. *Enzymes: The Fountain of Life.* Munich, Germany: Neville Press, Inc., 1994.

READING LIST

Ballentine, R. *Radical Healing.* New York: Harmony Books, 1999.

Barnard, N. *Foods That Fight Pain.* New York: Three Rivers Press, 1998.

Bock, K., and N. Sabin. *The Road to Immunity.* New York: Pocket Books, 1997.

Crook, W. *The Yeast Connection Handbook.* Berkeley, CA: Professional Books, 1999.

Cutler, E. W. *Winning the War Against Asthma and Allergies.* Albany, NY: Delmar Publishers, 1998.

D'Adamo, P. J. *Eat Right 4 Your Type.* New York: Putnam Publishing Group, 1997.

Daoust, J., and G. Daoust. *The Formula.* New York: Ballantine Books, 2001.

Gates, D. *The Body Ecology Diet,* 5th ed. Atlanta, GA: B.E.D. Publications, 1996.

Khalsa, D. S., and C. Stauth. *The Pain Cure.* New York: Warner Books, 2000.

Krohn, J., and F. Taylor. *Finding the Right Treatment.* Vancouver, Canada: Hartley & Marks Publishers, Inc., 1999.

Krohn, J., F. Taylor, and E. M. Larson. *Allergy Relief and Prevention,* 3rd ed. Vancouver, Canada: Hartley & Marks Publishers, Inc., 2000.

Lipski, E. *Digestive Wellness.* New York: Keats/NTC Contemporary, Inc., 2000.

Milne, R., and B. More, with B. Goldberg. *An Alternative Medicine Definitive Guide to Headaches.* Tiburon, CA: Future Medicine Publishing, Inc., 1997.

Murray, M. T. *Chronic Fatigue Syndrome.* Rocklin, CA: Prima Publishing, 1994.

Nichols, T., and N. Faass, eds. *Optimal Digestion.* New York: HarperCollins, 1999.

Northrop, C. *The Wisdom of Menopause.* New York: Bantam, Doubleday, Dell, 2001.

Ornish, D. *Dr. Dean Ornish's Program for Reversing Heart Disease.* New York: Ivy Books, 1996.

Pritikin, R. *The New Pritikin Program.* New York: Simon & Schuster, 1990.

Rogers, S. *Tired or Toxic?* Syracuse, NY: Prestige Publishing, 1990.

Saputo, L., and N. Faass, eds. *Boosting Immunity.* Novato, CA: New World Library, 2002.

Shames, R. *Thyroid Power.* New York: Harper Resource, 2001.

Steward, H., et al. *Sugar Busters.* New York: Ballantine Books, 1998.

WEB SITES

BIOSET™ INFORMATION

BioSET™ Institute of Dr. Ellen Cutler: includes information for consumers and health care professionals, practitioner referrals, and an on-line newsletter: www.bioset-institute.com

INFORMATION AND LINKS ON FOOD ALLERGIES

American College of Allergy, Asthma and Immunology: www.acaai.org

MEDICAL INFORMATION

National Institutes of Health article search: www.ncbi.nlm.nih.gov/PubMed/

Links to articles from the major medical journals: www.webmedlit.com

COMPLEMENTARY AND ALTERNATIVE MEDICINE

HealthWorld Online: www.healthy.com

National Center for Complementary and Alternative Medicine (NCCAM), an official NIH branch providing identification and evaluation of alternative health care practices: www.nccam.nih.gov/nccam/

The Richard and Hinda Rosenthal Center for Alternative/Complementary Medicine of Columbia University offers comprehensive information: cpmcnet.columbia.edu/dept/rosenthal/

Alternative Health News Online: www.altmedicine.com

RESOURCES

CONSUMER WORKSHOPS AND PROFESSIONAL SEMINARS

BioSET™ provides newsletters and information for the public and professionals, and referrals to practitioners trained in this method, as well as workshops and seminars.

The BioSET™ Institute
P. O. Box 7587
North Kansas City, MO 64116
Phone: (877) 927-0741
Fax: (415) 945-0465
Web site: www.bioset-institute.com
E-mail: admin@bioset-institute.com

ENZYME PRODUCTS AND DETOXIFICATION REMEDIES

Excellent quality vegetarian enzymes, homeopathic remedies for detoxification, empty glass vials, and copies of Dr. Cutler's books and video can be ordered through WellZymes at (800) 228-1501 or www.wellzymes.com

- The *Creating Wellness* videotape gives a clear, step-by-step demonstration of the BioSET™ Food Allergy Home Treatment described in Chapter 8.
- The BioSET™ Food Allergen Kit provides twenty-four vials containing over two hundred common food allergens. Empty vials are also available for preparing your own blood vial or for food allergens that are not provided in the kit.
- WellZymes Homeopathic Remedies for drainage, detoxification, energy production,

and specific organ support include Drainage, Detox, Recharge, Bladder Cleanse, Blood Cleanse, Colon Cleanse, Kidney Cleanse, Liver Cleanse, Lung Cleanse, Lymph Cleanse, Skin Cleanse, Small Intestine Cleanse, and Spleen Cleanse.

- WellZymes enzyme supplements for digestive health and systemic balance.
- The WellZymes Vitality Bar is the first energy bar enriched with plant-based enzymes. To learn more about this product, visit the WellZymes Web site at www.wellzymes.com, call (800) 228-1501, or pick up one of these energy bars at your neighborhood health food store.

HEALTH PRODUCTS AND RESOURCES

- Air and water filtration products: a comprehensive selection from Real Goods, a national catalog company

  www.realgoods.com or www.giam.com or www.gaiam.com

- Water filtration: filters and purification products appropriate for municipal or well water; whole-house treatment systems; consultations for problem water conditions, water testing, and show filters

  The Water Store
  184 Bon Aire Shopping Center
  Greenbrae, CA 94904

- Allergy supplies

  National Allergy Supply
  www.nationalallergysupply.com
  (800) 522-1448

- Back care: sleep and travel accessories, as well as ergonomically designed furniture, are available through the Back Store.

  www.relaxtheback.com
  (800) 290-2225

- Environmental Dental Association (EDA): information and referrals for the replacement of mercury fillings. For book orders, call EDA at (619) 586-7626. To receive a list of alternative dentists, send $3 and a self-addressed envelope stamped with 55¢ postage to:

  Environmental Dental Association
  P.O. Box 2184
  Rancho Santa Fe, CA 92067
  (800) 388-8124

- Genetically altered food:

  The Web site Greenpeace Guide lists thousands of everyday food products and whether they contain genetically altered ingredients.

  www.truefoodnow.org/shopping list

- Sauna

  Infrared Saunas
  Order number: (877) 839-0125
  Information at www.massageclinic.com

Index

ABOUT DR. ELLEN CUTLER

ELLEN W. CUTLER, M.D., D.C., holds medical and chiropractic degrees; she graduated with honors in both disciplines. She is a Diplomate of the National Board of Chiropractic Examiners and is board-eligible for Diplomate status with the American Board of Chiropractic Orthopedists. Her postgraduate training also includes nutrition, homeopathy, acupressure, and enzyme therapy. She continues to study intensively and conduct clinical research in the areas of immunology, nutrition, and allergy treatment.

Dr. Cutler is the developer and founder of BioSET™ (Bioenergetic Sensitivity and Enzyme Therapy), a highly effective system of healing. BioSET™ focuses on the treatment of allergy-related conditions, digestive disorders, immune dysfunction, and many other types of chronic illness. This treatment approach incorporates her knowledge of natural medicine and her clinical experience of more than twenty-five years in private practice, as owner and director of one of the largest complementary medicine centers in the United States.

A well-known author and media spokesperson, Dr. Cutler has written three books on the prevention and treatment of allergies and chronic health problems, including *Winning the War Against Asthma and Allergies* and *Winning the War Against Immune Disorders and Allergies;* she has also produced audiotapes on enzyme therapy, nutrition, and homeopathy, and a new video, *Creating Wellness.* She currently dedicates herself to teaching, writing, research, and the evaluation of patients with particularly complex conditions who come to see her from all over the world.